10 **THINGS I WISH I'D LEARNED** IN MEDICAL SCHOOL

A Practical Guide
to Sustainable Health

A.J. Seiffertt, D.O.

www.oneplanetonehealth.com

Edited by Heidi Mitchell

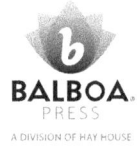

BALBOA
PRESS

A DIVISION OF HAY HOUSE

Balboa Press books may be ordered through booksellers or by contacting:

Balboa Press
A Division of Hay House
1663 Liberty Drive
Bloomington, IN 47403
www.balboapress.com
1 (877) 407-4847

Because of the dynamic nature of the Internet, any web addresses or links contained in this book may have changed since publication and may no longer be valid. The views expressed in this work are solely those of the author and do not necessarily reflect the views of the publisher, and the publisher hereby disclaims any responsibility for them.

The author of this book does not dispense medical advice or prescribe the use of any technique as a form of treatment for physical, emotional, or medical problems without the advice of a physician, either directly or indirectly. The intent of the author is only to offer information of a general nature to help you in your quest for emotional and spiritual well-being. In the event you use any of the information in this book for yourself, which is your constitutional right, the author and the publisher assume no responsibility for your actions.

The information, ideas, and suggestions in this book are not intended as a substitute for professional medical advice. Before following any suggestions contained in this book, you should consult your personal physician. Neither the author nor the publisher shall be liable or responsible for any loss or damage allegedly arising as a consequence of your use or application of any information or suggestions in this book.

Any people depicted in stock imagery provided by Getty Images are models, and such images are being used for illustrative purposes only. Certain stock imagery © Getty Images.

Print information available on the last page.

ISBN: 978-1-9822-2524-7 (sc)
ISBN: 978-1-9822-2526-1 (hc)
ISBN: 978-1-9822-2525-4 (e)

Library of Congress Control Number: 2019903945

Balboa Press rev. date: 04/22/2019

Thanks

To my editor, Heidi Mitchell, who is wonderful and thorough (and patient!) and brilliant (and kind!) and believed in this project straight away: I am so grateful for you. Thank you for your positive energy and excellent work.

To Larry and Linda, my first readers and biggest fans, who gave me much needed support early on and convinced me this was worth putting out into the world: Thank you!

To my friends and patients who kept asking me when this would be published: I am excited about finally handing you copies, and I appreciate your faith in me.

To my mom and grandfather, for your consistency and certainty that I was worth both listening to and arguing with: Thank you for the gifts of self-confidence and incredulity (we are from the "show-me-state" after all). I love you and miss you both so much. This book is dedicated to both of you.

CONTENTS

INTRODUCTION

This book is a compilation of the most helpful things I've learned since finishing medical school and residency: practices and concepts which have proved invaluable to my patients in the form of better health and better quality of life. Healing isn't simply the absence of illness or pain and is almost never instant. Healing is facilitated by carefully examining the conditions that give rise to your current state of health, and discovering what actions can be taken in order to remove the obstacles that are preventing your body from returning to its natural, balanced, optimal state of health. These ideas are helpful no matter what stage of life or health you find yourself in, whether you have just been diagnosed with cancer, a more chronic illness like diabetes, or simply don't feel as healthy as you might. Because living in greater health and peace *is* possible—no matter how many illnesses are plaguing you, and no matter how close you may be to death.

The key I have found comes in two parts. First, we need to make sure we understand when Western medications and treatments are necessary. Second, we need to know when evidence-based alternative approaches might do a better job over the long term, and how to implement them alongside Western treatments. These are things not currently taught—or at least not well—in most medical schools, and they are outright rejected in many.

When I first found myself in private practice, I discovered that most patients in the outpatient setting don't have the classic symptoms or disease processes that are described in medical textbooks. Attempting to work around patients' insurance (or lack of it), issues with access to care (or lack of it), and the side effects and cost of medications was frustrating for everyone. And because I often saw sparse results from the usual "best practices" I'd learned in school and residency, I became curious as to whether I could implement other methods of healing alongside the tools my training had given me. I wanted to find a way to practice a better form of medicine.

I spent years studying several "alternative" modalities outside my regular realm of practice, and started integrating this knowledge into my patient interviews and treatment plans. My earliest successes showed me the superiority of some of these concepts for reducing patient symptoms and the amount of medications necessary, for patients with issues ranging from pregnancy-related weight gain to brittle type 1 diabetes. Tailoring my treatment plans to individuals and building trusting relationships with my patients took time; it required working with them over months or years on their diet choices, exercise practices, and tapering or changing of medications. I learned that of the 80 percent of general practice patients who have chronic lifestyle diseases, many of them can reduce dependence on medications and begin to heal themselves—but they need a great deal of support with very good medical supervision, practical straightforward advice given in manageable doses, and encouragement. Essential for success is persistence and excellent communication in the challenging work done by both patient and doctor.

When I started this project, I intended nothing more than to write down the things I wish I had learned in medical school but had to learn on my own through successes with patients and extra post-residency schooling. The reason I continued writing this book was to communicate the vision shared by my patients and fellow practitioners who understand the interconnectedness of all things: whole person and whole planet health.

I am continually inspired by my patients, many of whom have had trouble navigating both alternative and modern medicine but have persisted and are learning to create conditions for their own improved health. I am also inspired by the hardworking scientists and advocates in the social justice and environmental movements, and would like to provide a bridge for people to understand how our own health is inextricably linked to the planet's health, right alongside social and economic justice. The changes I am working toward all intersect: social justice, health justice, environmental justice, and economic justice.

At least 60 percent of the determinants of health are economic and social factors; the medical system needs to take these factors into account and work with social and economic justice movements to fix the structural problems that make and keep people sick. Racial and economic disparities are direct causes of poor health and correlate with the worst areas of environmental pollution and toxic agricultural exposures. The trauma experienced by whole segments of our population, including refugees and immigrants who have an even harder time navigating our medical system because of language barriers, makes people sicker and is not taken into consideration by most of our medical system. When we know that a black trans woman's life expectancy is only around 35 years, it's even easier to see the direct harm injustice causes our patients. The medical community needs to be more aware, more vocal, and politically involved; we all need to work inside the system to remedy the structural problems that lead to people's ill health. We must integrate these concepts into the practice of medicine.

We know our bodies are not separate from our minds or our spiritual selves; we are not separate from each other; and we are not separate from the soil and air and water we depend on for survival. We aren't even separate from the animals and plants and fungi that share our home—we can't live without them. Our microbiome, living in and on us, proves that beyond any doubt. We can no longer behave as though we are a species apart, looking to technology or other planets to save us. It is irresponsible and absurd to continue looking to the far future with blind hope that "things will be okay," while we poison our water, our air, our soil, and ourselves. We had no idea what we were doing in ages past. Now that we have more than an inkling, there is no excuse for continued destructive behavior.

No matter what the establishment says or what your personal opinions are, the most sustainable ways to globally improve health involve finding ways to let the body heal itself with less financial cost, using the least possible pharmacological interventions, learning and practicing compassion across all social and economic strata, and taking the time to do it gently so the whole system (including individual human and global systems) can adapt and strengthen. This book is an introductory guide to the simplest of these principles.

In a nutshell, this book is about Sustainable Medicine: how we practice medicine today in the West is not sustainable for our planet's future any more than it is proving to be for the future health of our society. In the long run, patients are served better by having more time during appointments and being given individualized, thorough, and flexible care plans. Health improves and people are empowered when they don't need to rely on medications so heavily to treat chronic illnesses, and when they have doctors who are comfortable using any successful treatment from placebo to surgery.

I have seen that most chronic diseases can be slowed if not outright reversed with excellent care and persistence—which in our current system is a radical and disregarded notion. What I do is evidence-based, changes suggested are gradual, fads and expensive supplements are off the table, and the overriding idea is that the body will heal itself if allowed; it's a matter of figuring out what is preventing it from doing so and if these things are changeable. I am endlessly hopeful that everyone can have better quality of life, and I believe we can accomplish that without harming the world around us.

Here are several ideas that help me stay focused on bringing positive change to the practice of medicine:

- We in the medical field can expand our goals from defining success by symptom management and improved lab values to actually slowing and reversing chronic disease.
- We can help patients feel at peace and more in control of the most important parts of their lives, and we can feel more connected to and understanding of each patient we see.
- Doctors do not need to become more and more overwhelmed while patients feel more stuck, more sick, and more dependent on technology to save them.
- It is possible to teach doctors better ways of communicating with patients, and how to use information gained from a detailed history to help patients make gradual changes in their lifestyles.
- It is possible to use Western medicine to gain enough time to be able to implement more subtle and gradual changes that can actually begin to stabilize and reverse chronic illnesses.
- It is possible for health care workers to hold on to compassion and to the intent to decrease suffering that brought most of us into practicing medicine in the first place.
- It is possible to connect healthier human lives with improved systems of agriculture, community business, and healthier surrounding ecosystems.
- It is possible to make choices for our health that help address larger issues like climate change and social justice—even if on a tiny scale at first.
- It is possible to define health as a truly connected human experience.

I want to help connect these dots and expand the possibilities currently imagined in the usual practice of medicine. This book gives an idea of what is possible, why it is possible, how beneficial new thinking can be, and how each of us can help bring about changes in individual health and in the practice of medicine itself. Each chapter includes some background and some suggestions for where a person can start looking at the state of their own health in that particular area.

The idea is that if people have enough information about the conditions that bring on better health, they can begin to identify those areas in which they could make small and incremental—but ultimately very beneficial—changes in routine or lifestyle that may allow their health to begin to improve. Trying some of the tips and ideas in this book will make the obstacles you face as well as your potential areas of success more evident. Armed with this experimental evidence, a visit to the doctor will be more efficient, more informed, and more successful for both doctor and patient.

The advice here is directed toward those in "first world" countries, where chronic disease is more of a public health concern than infection, war, or famine. Although the principles here can be used in every country and every situation, they are of most use when the emergencies that Western medicine excels at treating have already been dealt with, and when individuals have some control over their diet and lifestyle habits. This is not the case in most places in the world, but given the economic and cultural tendencies towards unlimited growth and emulating the way things are done in the "developed" world, if we can change how we do things by becoming more mindful and holistic in our practice of medicine here, then hopefully we will all be moving in a better direction.[1]

Throughout, I make strong connections between our health and the planet we live on. Given the number of variables in the human body, the ecology of our planet, and what people in the fields of both medicine and environmental science have discovered in the last couple decades, it is clear to me that the two things are truly inseparable. What I am introducing here is the practical application of the concept of Sustainable Medicine.

Sustainable by itself means "to be able to continue a behavior indefinitely." In an environmental context it is generally used to mean "supporting ecological balance," or "using natural resources without depleting them." Sustainability is an overused term at this point, but there isn't a better word I've found for what I mean by it. One of the ways to think of it in an environmental context is "using natural resources without depleting them while healing prior damage, and while ensuring future generations can also use the resources." This is closest to the connotative and denotative meaning I'm going for when I came up with the phrases "sustainable medicine" and "sustainable health" a few years ago, although others have used these as well with different meanings and contexts.[2][3] A discussion and synthesis of the philosophy, ethics, science, and government policy involved is for my next book!

Useful definitions for this book:

Sustainable Health: ways to continue living within the web of our human community and our planetary ecology that heals prior damage, while ensuring our most fulfilling individual lives and the lives of our children and this planet centuries from now.

Sustainable Medicine: a collection of pragmatic ways physicians and other health care practitioners can educate, practice, and work together with patients to promote Sustainable Health.

Every major shift starts with just a few people. There are excellent ways to start reconnecting ourselves with our home while keeping both it and ourselves safe and healthy for much longer, with less suffering and more happiness than we have at present. The following chapters will dive into a few evidenced-based ways to start this process both at home and in the doctor's office. Then, in appendix 1, you will find "Sustainable Health Nutshells"— brief reminders of the basic sustainable health principles. I hope this book will encourage discussion and change within the medical profession itself and as to how we as a global community approach healing.

Please enjoy, and keep asking questions.

A.J. Seiffertt, D.O. 1/26/19

1

SUSTAINABLE MEDICINE:
AN OVERVIEW

We are living on a piece of solid and molten rock, suspended in a quiet void, a perfect distance from a ball of nuclear fusion that keeps everything on our rock at a temperature that doesn't kill us instantly. Our ball of molten and solid rock holds itself together—and holds onto the surface bits like us—with invisible forces, helped not just by its mass but also by the spinning that draws everything in and out at the same time. The atoms of the atmosphere, the water in the oceans, and the corn growing in Iowa, are all held in place gently by gravity. That ball of nuclear fusion gives us light and heat, and combined with the spin of our rock, regulates all the daily biorhythms of every plant and animal on the planet. Our moon, a gigantic rock itself, is slowly leaving us, extending its already faraway orbit, but for now it pulls the tides of our oceans and regulates all the monthly biorhythms of plants and animals.

This story is bonkers enough. Now think of atoms. Shrink yourself down to the size of an electron in an atom, with more than one of you in orbit of its nucleus. As an electron, you fly around a huge rock made of protons, neutrons, and maybe other things, with other electrons in different orbits, all held in place and kept spinning by invisible forces. As a whole, the system of this atom is 99 percent space. Maybe your atom is next to more atoms, and you make up a molecule—all held together by invisible forces. Maybe this molecule is located inside a cell.

The cell might have a nucleus too, around which float a sea of molecules and groups of molecules organized into organelles, held together by fluid but also by invisible forces. Maybe this cell is floating in an animal's bloodstream, or maybe it is less mobile and is linked to other cells in an organ. All the organs are connected to the blood stream and lymph channels and nerves, and the whole system is secured and contained by fascia and skin. But since every organ is made up of cells, and every cell is made up of molecules, and every molecule is made up of atoms, the entire system of a body that seems so solid and real is actually 99 percent space—like our galaxy, and the universe, too, if you'd like to zoom out that far.

These invisible forces include gravity and electromagnetic fields and many other forces we haven't become aware of yet. These forces also facilitate communication: in our own bodies between cells and organs, and among the animals and plants with which we share this home. Nothing exists in isolation, and invisible communication is occurring at every moment. We know that the small ways we communicate even non-verbally with others can change our own health and others' health. We know the small decisions we make affect our own health and also the health of other humans, and the consequences radiate out into our air and water and soil, affecting the whole of the ecosystem.

We are under the illusion that the reality we see with our five basic senses is constant. This illusion causes more illusions, like that our body is separate from our minds, or diseases in one part of the body aren't simultaneously affecting every other part of the body. We underestimate the effects of even one persistent negative thought on our immune system. We underestimate how love, compassion, and time in nature change our brains and health and affect everyone around us, radiating out in waves to the rest of the world and beyond.

We know we barely know anything about the how and why of our existence. But what we do know is that helping others and making healthy decisions for ourselves makes us feel good. We know that when we feel good and have enough energy for compassion and thinking outside ourselves, we can affect positive change in the world around us. We accumulate more and more knowledge every day about how we can make our home planet safer, cleaner, and more full of life. We need to add that to our knowledge of what makes us healthier individually and start changing the way we see human health and human medicine. We, as individual patients, working with health care practitioners of all kinds, can revolutionize medicine to promote true healing for both people and the planet.

To accomplish this medical revolution, we need to fully internalize and understand that there is no way forward—there are no healthy future generations—without a healthy environment. Doctors like me are in an excellent position to connect knowledge to practice and can make huge changes at the level of the individual that end up being cultural. Doctors and nurses at the front lines of health care have the capacity to be natural bridges between the shifting foundation of science and the practical application of our experience with thousands of individual patients. Our best function is to be teachers and guides, rather than dictators or medication dispensers.

The solutions to be looked for in the application of Sustainable Medicine are not just "science" or "alternative" or "environmental." There is no magic bullet. But there are small things that, if done every day, by everyone, can lead to huge positive change. Healing at this point in human evolution will require 50 percent science— "good science" though, science that includes outcome measures and individual variables in the research. The other 50 percent is about recognizing our humanness, grounded in the earth we come from, acknowledging human triumphs as well as mistakes made, and constantly reconnecting ourselves to the planetary rhythms and biological systems we've tried so hard to separate from—to our detriment and the detriment of the world around us.

This "other" 50 percent of Sustainable Medicine is about being fully human or, more accurately, *learning* to be fully human, since many of the activities we inflict on each other and the world are not what any of us would want to be remembered for. This includes learning from science and, looking forward, putting it all together so we can heal ourselves and the planet we harm so terribly every day. Being human means we can learn to be friendly and kind to our home that is also the only reason we are alive. We can be both caretakers and grateful neighbors to our planet—and our bodies.

There are outstanding examples of ways in which Sustainable Medicine has already made inroads into traditional medicine and thinking (although without being called Sustainable Medicine most of the time). Tying our personal health decisions to the health of the environment can be much simpler than we might think, and the "virtuous cycles" (as opposed to the vicious cycles we're maybe more familiar with) types of actions we can create in our environment are self-sustaining and deeply personally satisfying.[4] From "inner pharmacy hacks" like resetting our circadian rhythm, to reassessing cultural beliefs like "I can't call in sick for work," to avoiding too many antibiotic prescriptions, there are very simple things we can do that can improve everyone's life exponentially.

For doctors, models like direct primary care (monthly, subscription-based, primary care-only clinics that give unlimited time with your doctor and discounted services like lab work and x-rays), house-call doctor services, and so-called concierge medicine are all working to help GPs and internists have more time with patients and more time for themselves, while costing patients less in some cases. Even better, a single payer healthcare system would *save* money, like it does in other countries, especially if we can improve on existing models. Community health organizations like the one I work for now are innovating and improving quality of care in leaps and bounds, driven by high need and scarce resources. If similar models continue to be proven successful, this signals a welcome change in how we practice medicine in general, and creates a huge opening for integrating more sustainable medicine practices independent of pressures from insurance and pharmaceutical companies. If universal health care or a variant is accomplished, there will be an even better chance that preventative and sustainable primary care interventions will not only be reimbursed but also preferentially required by a single insurer. There is much work to be done.

There has been a burst of research activity in the past decade surrounding climate change and how it is affecting human health, in addition to economic and geographical changes. Already, over one million people have been relocated from coastal areas and the number is expected to rise as managed retreat has become a necessity faster than anticipated.[5] From dermatological diseases to Ebola, habitat loss, massive-scale agriculture, and changing environments for animals and insects, all make it much more likely that outbreaks of many types of illnesses will be more common in the years to come.[6] The Zika virus may be the newest example of this, as well as a good illustration of how collaboration across national boundaries can help us understand and reduce the damage from such outbreaks.

The fact that scientists are realizing these connections and attempting to study them means that finding solutions is becoming more achievable. These kinds of findings give more weight to arguments about reducing human impact on the air, water, forests, and the few areas left which are as yet untouched directly by humans. Given that extremes of climate are already being felt, especially in coastal areas and places where people are forced to live with the worst consequences of first world countries' waste, attention from the medical establishment can't arrive too soon.

Good news on the agricultural front is that young farmers are adopting new and successful business models for small farms. In Iowa, farmers who used to buy into "Big Ag" theories of crop management are finding that "carbon farming" (farming in such a way to cause carbon to be deposited in the soil faster than conventional farming, reducing greenhouse gasses in the air) is not only doable, but also economically more viable, especially over time.[7][8] Some Iowan farmers are also combating the problems of standard monocrop farming by implementing "multi-species grazing" on open pasture, regenerating the land and benefiting the rural economy by increasing jobs in the local area. In California, in light of the recent drought, farmers have found success with dry-farming typically water-intensive crops like tomatoes, grapes, quinoa, and almonds using permaculture principles.[9]

Amish farmers have found success not only with organic methods, but even more truly sustainable farming solutions. A great quote in an *Atlantic* article regarding this was: "Organic is a negative process certification. You can do nothing to your field and become certified. In contrast, we focus on actively restoring the balance found in natural systems."[10] This is taking Sustainable Medicine and applying it to farming, or maybe I am taking regenerative agriculture ideas and applying them to medicine! Professional fishers are also finding ways to make sustainable fisheries profitable for the long term, while restoring ecosystems up to 40 years faster than projected.[11] Dealing sustainably with the commons of the deep ocean is difficult, but with better satellite tracking and accountability, it is increasingly possible.

There are signs the food system is picking up on these sustainable principles and seeing the benefits for both people and the environment. This is natural from my perspective, since we "vote with our forks" three times a day. The food system seems the easiest place to start with policies and research to see what works and what doesn't. Although I don't encourage the type of "conscious capitalism" advocated by huge companies like Whole Foods, I do advocate supporting local farmers and small businesses who promote sustainability in their practices, since their actions directly support economic and environmental justice in an economy still largely driven by profit that is dependent on externalizing costs and keeping the labor force oppressed. For example, Harvard University and the Culinary Institute of America recently came up with a simple set of guidelines for the food service industry (which pointedly left out suggestions for economic justice, but the food guidelines are decent).[12] A few key food and packaging additives that are likely toxic to humans have been banned by the FDA, thanks to the work of the Natural Resources Defense Council and the Environmental Working Group, and hopefully more attention will be paid to this area of research and regulation.[13]

In France, the successful grocery chain Day by Day uses no packaging at all, reducing food waste as well as packaging waste. Similar stores, like Granel in Spain, Unpackaged in the U.K., and in.gredients and Zero Market in the U.S., have also been successful in the past few years. *The Economist* and *The Guardian* have both reinforced the evidence-based benefit of greenhouse gas-lowering diets, arguing for reduced meat consumption, particularly processed meats, which are the most harmful from a health perspective, and red meats, which require more resources to produce and emit more carbon into the atmosphere.[14] [15] In January 2019, the journal *The Lancet* published a very helpful comprehensive report by the EAT-Lancet commission that outlines the ways those in both wealthy and poorer countries need to change their food systems and food consumption in order to improve human health and to make sure our consumption of resources is sustainable for our planet.[16]

Fortunately, obvious health choices that have been ignored because of industry lobbying are getting more publicity as well. A recent study found that children who are provided water instead of sugary drinks at school lose weight without other interventions, helping break their addictions to sugar and improving their health.[17] Added benefits of school policies supporting healthier choices is the inherent large-scale "voting" against companies and government policies that generate unhealthy and environmentally harmful products dependent on conventional agriculture.

Using institutions to implement sustainable practices is an excellent way to impact larger numbers of vulnerable populations, exemplified by the Intergenerational Learning Center at Providence Mount St. Vincent in Seattle, where children and the elderly help each other learn. A documentary called *Present Perfect* was recently made about this community, adding to the growing amount of research involving children, animals, and nature in nursing homes and schools that are improving health and quality of life, as well as adding to longevity. In Maine and elsewhere, medical residency programs are introducing food-centered education alongside traditional approaches to nutrition and illness treatment, in the hope that the programs become scalable examples that lifestyle medicine is both economically feasible and a valued part of everyone's health care. These types of models are noteworthy and heartening.[18]

Global population growth is important to address, since exponentially more resources seem to be needed for exponentially more people. But when education and health care—and specifically education and health care for women—is emphasized in countries with the largest population growth rates, birth rates drop precipitously. At the same time, women attain more freedom and control over their lives, making child raising more economically and emotionally feasible.[19] The availability of a variety of forms of birth control allows women to choose when and if they wish to have children, while reducing abortion and infanticide rates in poor and rich countries alike. Women who are educated and allowed to contribute to their families in ways they choose are more likely to become involved in politics, policy making, health care, and cultural enrichment in their communities. Women's rights have come to the forefront of many global discussions in the past decade, positively contributing to finding sustainable solutions to planetary health.

There are bright spots, too, in the research on how fast nature is able to bounce back from human interference if given the opportunity. In Olympic National Park in Washington, after a dam was removed, salmon returned and fish contributed to improved forest health faster than expected.[20] And although there are looming frights about rising temperatures letting loose the huge amount of carbon stored in permafrost, and how indigenous people are being harmed by mining, particularly in Canada and Brazil, with better global communication we are becoming more and more aware of the disasters as well as the apparent miracles happening around the world.[21] Global health is a huge field of study, and the complex sets of issues surrounding creating sustainable solutions around the world are being studied, and mistakes are being admitted.[22] [23] To me, these are also steps in a positive direction and bode well for our ability to adapt and survive without continuing to leave only destruction in our wake.

Sustainable Medicine is the necessary way to approach human health as we move into the future. Looking at the causes of death in the U.S. in 1990 and 2000, not much has changed: in 1990, eighty-five percent of the leading causes of death were preventable lifestyle causes and in 2000, ninety-three percent were.[24] From tobacco and alcohol to poor diet and exercise to motor vehicle accidents and firearms, the statistics show we are doing a poor job of improving our ability to reverse chronic disease and come up with policies to help us avoid risky behaviors.

We can do better, and we can do it in a sustainable way that is much more affordable. We can do it in a way that improves the health of patients and doctors, and helps take the stress and confusion out of the current medical system for both.[25] We can make the system more sustainable so that other countries around the world can implement similar changes without relying entirely on more pharmaceuticals or ever more expensive equipment. Alongside our commitment to enacting necessary policy changes, we can use Sustainable Medicine principles to guide our individual choices as physicians and as patients, to help the environment at the same time our choices help us.

In order to do this most effectively, doctors need more time with patients and to see fewer in a day. The current system is set up so that most doctors in outpatient primary care clinics, in order to pay malpractice and overhead as well as make a salary that will pay off medical school debt, must see patients in about 10-minutes, with no time for lunch or a break. The accompanying paperwork that is required keeps doctors at work, seated and glued to computer screens, well past when the last patient goes home. There is a growing shortage of primary care doctors and at the same time a growing surplus of patients in need of doctors, especially aging patients.

In the U.S., we have a ratio of about one primary care doctor to three specialists, but to be most efficient and catch diseases before specialists are needed, and to reverse chronic diseases and manage them more effectively, the ratio should be closer to one specialist to two primary care doctors. We need to reevaluate our dependence on specialist care, especially since some of the most expensive and typical interventions we've relied on for decades in specialties like cardiology may not actually improve outcomes.[26] We must start valuing primary care—including geriatrics, pediatrics, family practice, and internal medicine—as much as or more than we value specialties and procedures.

Equity and justice in the workplace must also be addressed, particularly in medicine where female physicians and physicians of color still earn less than male physicians for the same work. Many of those in positions of power still deny the existence of structural sexism and racism. Confronting and rectifying these issues in the medical field is an excellent way to promote social justice at a community level, since everyone comes in contact with a medical practitioner at some time or another.

If insurance companies and/or government programs start to reimburse primary care doctors more than the current standard and encourage doctors to take extra time with patients, more of our best doctors will choose to be primary care physicians. This is an essential piece of the puzzle of making medicine sustainable, since primary care physicians are THE front line workers. Doctors need to have more time to get to know patients better, we need to be valued for our breadth and depth of knowledge, and we need to have the freedom to work normal hours so we can have fulfilling lives outside of work, just like we recommend to our patients.

John Muir wrote in his journal in 1869: "When we try to pick out anything by itself we find that it is bound fast by a thousand invisible cords that cannot be broken, to everything else in the universe." Everything is part of a complex system, and this is especially apparent in the case of medicine. The human internal ecosystem and the external planetary ecosystem are so intertwined that there is no separation. We humans are good at learning and problem solving, and the solutions to problems of human health and the environment are frequently the same problems and can be solved together. We must focus our efforts on solutions and creativity, and use our intelligence to connect our hearts and minds back to the planet, since a healthy planet is the only way to ensure human survival.

It is not difficult to envision a future where we use the sun and wind and geological heat to fuel our technology, since in many countries green energy is overtaking fossil fuels already. It isn't difficult to imagine a future where we use sustainable farming methods across the globe instead of burning rainforests, where intact ecosystems are left alone to their beautiful devices, and where people are enabled by good policy to make healthful and sustainable lifestyle choices. With access to unlimited "green" energy resources and being able to rely primarily on locally sourced food, there will be fewer reasons for war.[27] In this kind of future there are more reasons for collaboration, and fewer reasons to disturb peace and our ability to understand each other.

I advocate strongly teaching simple Sustainable Health solutions to physicians and other health professionals, including in medical schools. And those of us out of training who are able to work on policy changes can help the system favor preventative and sustainable practices, like extended patient appointment times and reductions in medication necessity, and we can work to change the reimbursement ratio for specialists and primary care physicians. There is no reason besides inertia that these changes can't affect the next class of medical students and current practicing health care providers of all kinds. The only difference between what I've written here and what is already taught is a question of emphasis and amount of time spent helping students understand how to implement these techniques for individual patients.

And of course patients are the ones with the real power here. This collection of sustainable health principles can be used in two ways: 1) to evaluate how you are doing and find areas you might need help with, and 2) to start making changes in your health choices on your own. One of the main ideas behind Sustainable Medicine is that you know your body and your life best, so a better understanding of how your body functions with its natural healing mechanisms gives you more tools and insight to improve and maintain your own health. You can use these principles to troubleshoot and discover which of your personal obstacles to health are the hardest to remove and might require assistance. Knowing these principles also gives you more information to take to your doctor, whether you have health problems or simply want to work more efficiently to avoid them.

I often say that any advice in this book is to be discussed with your doctor before implementing it—this is to make sure your health plan is individualized and monitored in person by someone who knows you. If you don't have a primary care doctor, then that is tough. You might not like Western medicine, or maybe had a doctor you liked long ago but they retired and you haven't found one you trust since. If you're in a big healthcare system, you may see a different doctor, Physician's Assistant, or Nurse Practitioner every time you go in; they can see your overall chart but may not know you well. They can still give general advice based on your history, however, and that will suffice for what I advise in this book.

If you don't have a Western doctor, I suggest you find a way to see one, just to make sure nothing obvious is being missed; screening for things best caught early like cervical cancer, diabetes, and other illnesses is important. Symptoms of fatigue or feeling unwell should be checked out, and you want to make sure you're safe when embarking on a new food or exercise program. If finances are a problem, Planned Parenthood, community health centers (sometimes called Federally Qualified Health Centers, because they receive funding to reduce costs for patients), Tribal Health clinics, and VA systems do a really good job of the basics, and they have the most affordable options for those with little or no insurance. Until we have a better health system in this country, it will continue to be a struggle for many of us to have adequate care, so I need to stress the obvious—this book isn't a substitute for individual medical care or personal advice. Please use caution and good judgment for your own individual medical needs, and only use this book as a guide.

Changing how we think about medicine, what is emphasized in medical school, and how we practice won't happen overnight, but the principles of Sustainable Medicine are universally applicable and helpful around the globe. There are no arguments against any of the simplest interventions, and evidence is building for even the most multifaceted principles, such as caring for our personal microbiome by supporting increased diversity, and cultivating our epigenetic potential with excellent lifestyle choices.[28] When even our most prestigious universities start advocating nature as one of "life's best anti-inflammatories," we are well on our way to a paradigm shift towards Sustainable Medicine.[29]

2

WHAT HEALS YOU?

Practicing medicine the "slow" way is the only sustainable way to move forward.

The term *healer*, while having an appeal, worries me. It gives more power to a person outside oneself than is warranted by the specific skill set and knowledge of a physician or nurse. While I do know of people with seemingly miraculous talents for accurate diagnosis or who have great success in some cases with their treatments of choice, I've never seen someone actually "heal" another person. Any healing accomplished is actually done by the body in need of the healing. Healing occurs when the impediments to normal functioning are removed, and the inherent systems of health are allowed to flourish, build, and repair correctly. It is a matter of the body shifting itself from disequilibrium to equilibrium—or what science terms homeostasis.

Whether it is eradication of bacteria, restoration of broken tissue from accident or surgery, hormonal rebalancing, or for those who believe in energy fields, realigning those fields or restoring the flow, the body's systems, cells, and internal communications perform the healing. Outside forces might assist by killing a majority of pathogenic organisms or cancer cells, by physically removing a malfunctioning organ, or keeping a shattered bone in alignment with temporary screws and pins. But in the end, the immune system is responsible for finishing off the remaining pathogens or cancer cells, and the body's repair cells restore tissue damaged by infection or trauma, including the trauma of the surgeon's knife. No matter how perfect the stitches after a surgery, whether health returns to the body is not up to the physician, the medicine, or even the patient's conscious mind.

This lack of power to directly affect illness is difficult for humans to bear, and over the eons, we've turned to each other, gods, and the earth around us for help. Over time, "medicine people" were identified as having special insight or skill in dealing with illness, physical or spiritual. These practitioners used anything within reach to assist in bringing a patient back to health, or at the very least to provide some comfort and peace. Until relatively recently, doctors were able to tell when they had done what they could, and when to leave the rest up to fate, a god, or the ill patient themself. But in the last hundred years, technology has improved so vastly that it seems physicians and nurses actually do have the power to heal—or at least they can depend on miraculous technology to fix any problem.

Unfortunately, the incredible advances in science that have led to more accurate diagnosis and treatment, and magnificently improved medicines and surgical techniques, have pushed us in the direction of appearing to have more omniscience than we actually possess. At the same time, our reliance on science has caused us to overlook time and again some of the most obvious mechanisms by which the body heals itself, missing opportunities to avoid the need for quite so much technology and medicine.

During my third year of medical school, while interviewing some of my earliest "real" patients, I remember how frantically I tried to remember all the questions I needed to ask. As med students, we were drilled in information gathering; we learned how to elicit useful facts and made sure we wrote every detail down. Over time, we were expected to grow more efficient at knowing what was vital and what was irrelevant. We asked about medicines, allergies, medical history, family and social history, pain location, duration, and quality, and the lengthy "review of systems"—all while trying to let the patient speak enough to tell us their "chief complaint" and "history of present illness," so we could write it down to present to the attending physician. It was always embarrassing to learn I'd missed something when the attending came to interview the patient, and through my panic I tried to appear calm and knowledgeable when the person was speaking, while not rushing them or taking too long with my side of the interview.

I know I looked foolish, trying to look up to make eye contact and nod, then back down to write, then pausing and staring into space to remember my questions… I'm sure I looked very young to the patients who were kind enough to let me learn on their time and from their troubled health. In the years since, two glaring omissions in my early patient interviews have become apparent. The first is a common mantra of professors in medicine: listen long enough and the patient will tell you the diagnosis and treatment. The reality is that sometimes listening can be better medicine than medicine.

The second important question I had to learn for myself is, "What heals you?" Variations and related questions could be: "When do you feel your best? When did you last feel really healthy, and what was your life like then? What has changed?" And depending upon the answers received, the job of a physician arises: "Given the reality of life now, with whatever limitations are real or perceived, what can we do together to get you moving towards health once again?"

Modern Medicine's Blind Spots

Thinking carefully about how we practice medicine these days, it is clear that medicines and surgeries don't actually heal anything. If capillaries did not clamp down and allow blood-clotting mechanisms to stop the flow, everyone would bleed to death after a bad hangnail. If cells that were sliced or cauterized during surgery were not removed by immune cells and rapidly replaced by new cells bridging the gap held together by the stiches, everyone who underwent intestinal surgery would die within hours. Cancers are largely an example of backup system breakdown, where the immune system and normal programmed cell death both fail, and treating it (in almost all cases until recently) involves inflicting dramatic traumas from which we hope the system can recover, this time cancer-free.

While the old tenet *anything is a poison or a health tonic, depending on dose* is indeed true, many medicines such as antibiotics and chemotherapy function as direct poisons, albeit targeted ones. We hope they leave enough "good" cells alive to let the person's immune system recover. The side effect lists from most medicines on the market are frightening, sometimes seeming worse than the illness they are designed to treat. This can be a brutal way of going about facilitating healing, even as miraculous healing often results from their administration.

And, as is the case with most medicines that are in theory my "bread and butter" as an internal medicine doctor, the medicines themselves don't improve the illnesses at all. Types of medicines that lower blood pressure, blood sugar, cholesterol, and regulate hormones only work to stabilize or add a missing function to a body that is not working well. We can think of most of these treatments as treating symptoms, whether silent and in need of technology to notice them (like high blood sugar or blood pressure) or obvious to the patient (like diabetic neuropathy pain or gout). These medicines are important, of course, and add years to people's lives that would otherwise be shortened significantly by their illnesses. Some of them do help incrementally with things like cholesterol plaque reduction and heart muscle remodeling. Significantly, most of these medicines only help as long as they are taken regularly. Few do very much to repair the underlying damage created by the imbalanced systems that caused the symptom the medicines attempt to dampen, and when the drugs are stopped, symptoms usually return and can temporarily rebound worse than before the medication was begun.

For example, if you forget a day of blood pressure pills, the upward swing in blood pressure that results in the next day or so is more dangerous than having slightly high blood pressure for months. If you are a diabetic and forget your blood sugar medicine or accidentally take an extra dose, a resulting diabetic emergency can send you to the hospital. Suddenly stopping a statin medication for cholesterol can result in a temporarily increased risk for heart attack, due likely to a rebound effect in the inflammatory pathway the medication tamps down. Thyroid medication, for those whose thyroid gland no longer functions, needs to be monitored frequently. Too much or too little can result in huge metabolic problems that come on so gradually they might be passed off as depression, a bit of weight gain or loss, fatigue or stress, or increasing blood pressure and heart disease.

Many medications deplete certain necessary vitamins as well, adding to potential side effects. Many doctors are unfamiliar with these common nutrient deficits, and we don't yet know the most effective ways of adding these nutrients to the diets of patients who take these medications. The usual assumed treatment is to add supplements to the diet, or to restrict certain foods, but very little research has been done to deem these interventions effective and beneficial for overall health, longevity, or side-effect elimination.

Overall in our Western medical culture, we tend to think of chronic illnesses like heart disease and diabetes as permanent diagnoses. If we diagnose someone with one of these in the clinic or hospital, we remind patients that "losing weight" and eating "healthier" can improve lab values associated with these problems. Health practitioners frequently use shame or logical admonishments to motivate patients to "change their lifestyles," but neither party usually believes it is possible—even though research proves that genetically high-risk patients can reduce their risk by 50 percent with the smallest of lifestyle changes.[30] [31] The assumptions are that the health of everyone deteriorates with age, genetic predispositions to chronic diseases are not modifiable, and insistence on eating the "standard American diet" is too difficult to change. And since the main concern is always making sure the patient stays "stable" and out of the hospital (and alive), the least complicated way we health practitioners know to accomplish this is to prescribe pills.

The medications on the market, if taken as directed and monitored frequently, often do an adequate job of keeping chronic disease patients' systems stable. They reduce risk of heart attack, stroke, and organ damage, and extend patients' lives significantly. But they don't cure. They don't reverse the disease process very much. And maybe worst of all, they add to a general culture of depending on a simple external miracle to keep us alive, while taking away our hope of having the power to improve our own health. The tools of medicines and surgery don't teach patients about the body or health, nor can those tools listen to our stories about how we got where we are and what is most important to us in our lives.

Healing Takes Time

The truth of why the system has failed chronic disease patients (and many others) is simple. Healing at nature's speed, rather than miraculous speed, takes time. Every single chronic or "lifestyle" disease someone is suffering from developed over a period of years, and even acute illnesses very often happen because the body is already chronically stressed in some way. Over time, many components of the body's systems have changed to compensate for both environmental and genetic factors. Every time a choice is made that is hard on the body, whether it is dietary, lifestyle, work, or family related, the body responds and tries to balance it with a reaction to keep the system's precarious balance steady.

This has been necessary throughout human evolution. If we didn't raise our blood pressure to run from predators or to hunt them, we might either be eaten or just not have food to eat. When we found an abundance of one type of food and ate a lot of it, our systems accommodated it and our gut bacteria changed rapidly to get us the most nutrition and energy from the new food. Our bodies are unbelievably flexible and miraculously adaptable to what we present them with—to a point.

If we continually make choices that require compensation, our body's responses stiffen and become stuck. Too little sleep, ongoing rather than temporary stress, eating large amounts of simple carbohydrates and oxidized fats, all take their toll on multiple organ systems at once. Kidney, liver, and pancreatic functions change and weaken, receptors for hormones are down- or up-regulated, microbial diversity plummets, our immune system suffers, artery walls become thickened to accommodate chronic higher pressures, inflammation increases as abdominal fat increases, muscle and fat tissue respond less to sugar in the blood stream... while the ability to easily reverse these changes retreats from our grasp.

There was a bit of a blame-game debate in the science community a couple of years ago over whether cancers are "accidents" of genetics or whether environmental and behavioral effects are more responsible. A group from Johns Hopkins found that around two thirds of cancers are from genetic malfunctions.[32] They used the analogy of a car with bad brakes trying to take a long journey, saying that if your car was faulty, your chances of accident are higher and likely inevitable. They acknowledged the many variables involved, but were very certain in their conclusions. Eleven months later, another study came from Stonybrook University's statistics department, which showed 70 to 90 percent of cancers have environmental triggers. This means around 30 percent of cancer is at least partially preventable. That's quite something.

Both studies have merit and issues (lack of racial and gender diversity in these studies is a huge, common, and recurrent problem with much of today's research). We already know from epigenetic research on many types of cancers and other genetically linked illnesses that environmental and personal behavior can turn genes on and off.[33] [34] [35] [36] And we know from the newest microbiome research that our bacterial friends in our guts help turn genes on and off: we depend on their diversity and health for our own health. It would be convenient if most cancers have a purely genetic basis, since it might make research for cures simpler. The reality is, however, that our behavior choices play a huge role in how our body heals and responds to its environment and its own genetic predispositions.

My favorite part of some of the recent studies is that relatively simple lifestyle changes make huge differences in risk.

- Not smoking or having stopped five years back
- Being less than obese but not thin
- Exercising a moderate amount of time weekly
- Drinking less than one drink a day for women, less than two for men

Doing all four of these cuts risk for cancer and heart disease in half—that's better than most medications. Making even more healthy lifestyle choices goes even further. This should give those of us with family history some hope, and those of us with a past of not-so-healthy behaviors incentive that small changes can make a huge difference.

Lifestyle Changes Are Key and Possible

When illness does happen, yes, medicines can force blood pressure down and stave off artery, heart, nerve, and kidney damage. Yes, medicines can do an adequate job of reducing blood sugar and improving its uptake. And yes, we can help many people with chronic illnesses control their symptoms and live much, much longer than ever before. But there is no pill that will fix the underlying cause of chronically high blood pressure or the underlying cause of type II diabetes, or of anything else. Yes, advances in genetic and immune therapies are exciting and mean we may be able to actually *cure* certain illnesses, especially those that have clear genetic causes, which would be welcome and truly miraculous.[37] But it is unlikely that we will find magic cures to resolve decades of poor health choices, and sometimes genetic predisposition is too powerful to reverse, especially after decades of stress. Time and again, research shows that chronic conditions are best managed with minimal medication and a solid foundation of optimized individualized lifestyle behaviors.

We know that changes in lifestyle *do* cure many chronic diseases. We know that in many cases a strict diet can dramatically reduce cholesterol deposits in arteries that increase heart attack risk, and cholesterol pills cannot. We know exercise reduces insulin resistance and that weight loss can eliminate the need for blood pressure and/or diabetes medications and asthma treatments in some people whose diseases are caused primarily by their lifestyle. Even in patients whose genetic background makes them much more likely to develop these problems, despite good diet and exercise, an individualized diet, exercise, and stress reduction plan can do wonders in reducing medication requirements and can improve their lives far beyond only lab values. We each have a massive "inner pharmacy" in our brains and GI tracts which, when allowed adequate sleep, sunlight, exercise, and healthful whole foods, functions better than most medications to help our bodies have enough energy and resources to prevent illness and fight disease.

There Is No Age Limit on Healing: Polly

When healing is defined as improving the quality of life, this means that anyone can heal. No disease is too serious or close to the end of life that a more holistic way of practicing medicine won't help. The extent of healing can simply be providing some peace and freedom from suffering all the way to reversing illnesses entirely. Although some illnesses that have been established for years may take nearly as many years to reverse, remarkably, sometimes the timeline to cure is far shorter than anyone would expect, even in older patients.

One patient I particularly enjoyed working with was a woman in her eighties. I'll call her Polly here, and combine a bit of her story with other patients' to protect her personal information. She came to me with diagnoses of high blood pressure, weight gain, decreased ability to exercise due to arthritis, and back problems including scoliosis. When we met, I found her to be a bit overweight and to have kidneys only functioning around 30 percent. She had a fall a few years back, and had been diagnosed with arthritis instead of a fracture, for which she was given anti-inflammatory pain medicine. At the same visit, she was also diagnosed with high blood pressure for which she was given first one, then two blood pressure medications to reduce her risk of stroke and heart problems, and to rid her of some leg swelling that had worsened.

A few months after her injury, Polly saw another doctor

that diagnosed her with a "partially healed fracture" rather than arthritis and had her work with physical therapy. She compensated well over the next few years, despite the frustration of not understanding what happened with her first diagnosis, and she tried various therapies to help her exercise more with small success. Soon after, she ended up moving nearer to her children, very much missed her old doctor, and like anyone would be, was wary of medicines and doctors she didn't know well.

When Polly came to see me, cautious and very clear about what she needed from me, it took a while to get to know her. I obtained her previous medical records and reviewed them in detail since her medication list didn't make sense to me. Looking at the timeline I'd made for myself with her lab values, I found that her new diagnosis of chronic kidney disease coincided exactly with her fall and subsequent medication additions. Anti-inflammatory pain medicines can cause problems with kidneys when blood pressure is too high or too low, especially in the elderly, so I wondered why she had been kept on that medicine when her kidney function was poor. We also found over a few months of visits to my office that pain and anxiety raised her blood pressure despite the two medications she was on, but when she was at home and relaxed, her pressure sometimes dropped dangerously low.

Over a few months of osteopathic manipulation visits and regular appointments to track her progress, we found a different pain medicine that affected the kidneys less that she could take if needed. I also slowly reduced and removed her blood pressure medicines, adding back a tiny dose of a diuretic occasionally for her chronic leg swelling. Her blood pressure barely changed, but her bouts of too-low blood pressure went away, and it ended up remaining within acceptable limits for her age and risk profile with no medicines at all.

We spent a good deal of time discussing her diet and hydration status. She started drinking more water during the day and found healthier foods that appealed to her. Over the few years we worked together, Polly lost weight, reduced her rising blood sugar, and exercised more. We had troubleshooting issues sometimes, and life's stresses occasionally derailed a bit of progress, but overall, her health, and her understanding of it, was much better. In addition, her willingness to learn to meditate and practice stress-reducing techniques helped her tremendously, especially when her partner developed frightening and frustrating health problems of his own.

The most medically surprising thing about Polly's story was that after removing the kidney-offending medications, her kidney function returned to normal. I had never seen or expected someone of her age who had had poor kidney function for over three years improve to a value that was normal even for someone younger. As a case study it made logical sense, but it still went against common assumptions about the progression of kidney disease and how much plasticity older bodies have. It was another reminder to me that by taking adequate time, more kinds of healing are possible than we imagine in our day-to-day practices. No matter a person's age or medical issues, healing is always possible.

Successful Treatment Plans Take Communication and Patience

Two things you will notice from Polly's story are that individualizing treatment takes time, and mostly what was done was removing obstacles to healing. Finding out what lifestyle and medication changes will actually stick takes time. It needs both doctor and patient continually working on communication to learn to understand each other well. It takes trial and error over multiple visits to find out together which diet or specific foods will work. It also takes troubleshooting age, medical problems, and injuries to find out what type of exercise is enjoyable enough to do regularly over the long term.

It might take even longer to develop the trust that allows

you to discuss stress, relationships, family, and culture, and what larger lifestyle adjustments might be possible. As a patient, it is important to be open to these discussions and to be willing to self-evaluate and do small experiments on your own to find what foods, exercise, or other lifestyle changes you might be able to keep up and enjoy. For doctors, it's important to make the time to do this kind of deep listening and problem solving from our perspective of wider experience and medical knowledge.

What allowed my patient's kidneys to heal was removing the offending medications, keeping her from getting dehydrated, and giving them stress-free time to heal. This is the same principle used by ecologists to restore ecosystems, and it often works better and faster than any direct intervention. Above all, allowing healing requires imagination and patience and truly attempting to understand the patient's world. The biggest obstacle from my perspective as a physician is that none of us learn *how* to do this in medical school or residency.

A couple of years ago I was looking into going back to teaching, and I was hoping to integrate some of the ideas in this book into my classes. But the mantra I heard from medical school education directors, residency programs, and most physicians was dismissive of holistic approaches to healing. It boiled down to: "We must focus on getting the science and medicine details right; there is time for nothing else." I understand that for medical school deans, the goal of medical education is to have the largest number of students possible pass their board exams and get into residency programs. This ensures the students know enough science to be ready for residency. It also makes the numbers look good and allows the school to attract more students—tuition from these students is the lifeblood of a university. The way our education system is set up, there's nothing wrong with this, and I might have had similar priorities if I were in their shoes. I fully support the amazing science that has given us extended life spans and the ability to recover from what used to be life-threatening problems, and of course medical students need to learn all of that.

What I disagree with in the current system is the automatic and reflexive idea that follows this heavy emphasis on learning the hard science: that there is always more time for more science, but no time to spend on teaching what is usually referred to as "integrative medicine." What I call integrative medicine broadly means taking time to get to know patients and prescribing only absolutely necessary medications, mostly to buy time. We then use that time to our best advantage to work on reversing the disease process by correcting the underlying causes of the imbalances that led to the disease. We constantly review medication lists and make sure they are minimal and optimal as each patient's health changes. Reversing disease requires creativity, patience, and innovative methods personalized to each patient. It requires physicians to know more than they are currently taught in most medical schools and residencies.

I need to reiterate here that this is not alternative or complementary medicine—this is "real medicine." It is closer to what medicine aspires to be than what it now looks like to patients and doctors 90 percent of the time: namely, treating lab numbers and symptoms primarily with pills, with doctors spending two thirds of their time on documentation and administrative tasks. What the best physicians do is facilitate a simple process: they listen to the patient, then both patient and doctor agree on a plan to remove obstacles to good health, with medicines and other methods, and then everyone crosses their fingers while waiting to see if healing will take place or not. If it does, they take the next steps closer to health, and if it doesn't, there is now information available from the failure of the first plan to do better on the next try.

Medicine in its true sense is more than just the science; it is an art and practice, and art and practice take time. Insurance companies and research guidelines encourage us to be satisfied with symptom and number management, even though we know there are ways to help patients heal more fully. We are encouraged to pack in as many patients as possible, and the fee structures reinforced by insurance companies reflect this and cause doctors to work longer hours and see more patients with shorter appointment times. Procedures with immediate results are rewarded, and time spent with patients to prevent disease and procedures is not. The current system makes many physicians yearn to be able to do better, causes many to burn out and quit medicine entirely, and some of us are driven to work towards changes that will allow us to do better.

Doing better requires knowledge of nutrition and diet modifications that are flexible and can be changed to work in different cultural scenarios and genetic backgrounds. It requires familiarity with different types of exercise that can be modified for age and ability and injury. It means knowing how to advise patients on sleep optimization and daily routines that are nourishing and allow the body time to heal. It also requires being able to apply counseling and stress-reduction techniques from multiple angles that will help patients prioritize and be better able to help themselves. These are the things that actually help bring the body back to an equilibrium where it can stop spending all its energy on compensating, and instead can begin self-repair, self-regulation, and more efficient use of energy.

When the body's systems come closer to balance, a person is more likely to feel healthy and have the energy to meet life's challenges. Patients can learn what heals them, and we can help with both our knowledge of science and also with our experience and patience. THAT is *medicine*. It is sustainable medicine. It promotes healing and reverses the worldwide trends of increasing chronic disease and debility. It is not "integrative" or "alternative," but simple, necessary, medicine.

Changing How We Think About and Practice Medicine

So what can we do to change how we practice medicine as doctors but also as patients? How do we learn to better facilitate the body's healing? Teaching the *how* of these ideas to medical students and residents is necessary, but we must also find ways to work this type of "slow medicine" into our modern system. Proving it works on a large scale will be key to winning the financial arguments that keep general practice doctors seeing patients every seven to ten minutes. Thankfully, ideas like this are already in full swing with revolutionary movements like the push for single-payer healthcare, models of care with a team approach, like integrative medicine centers within Federally Qualified Health Centers, some versions of direct primary care, and projects like the Eden Alternative[38] [39] in Australia, Canada, the U.K., and the U.S., all of which provide useful statistics and financial success stories.[40] [41] The example of the midwife-centered program at Tuba City Hospital in Arizona, run by the Navajo Nation, illustrates how lower surgery rates and a different insurance and reimbursement model can vastly improve care.[42] It has also been shown that instead of criminalizing homelessness and drug abuse, simply giving the homeless homes and treating drug addiction as we would mental illness, while simultaneously focusing on support and community, can work better and be economically more practical.[43]

Since many modalities in Integrative Medicine are more affordable than those of Western medicine, and are already being used by indigenous and underserved communities, the Integrative Medicine for the Underserved (IM4US) conference was created in 2011. IM4US attempts to address issues of equity and justice in medicine. This group brings together doctors and other health care providers, and highlights community health clinics around the country that are doing excellent work with underserved patients, including children and refugees. A few of the model clinics are associated with large medical teaching centers such as Northwestern, Oregon Health & Science University, St. Louis University, and the University of Chicago. Others are in underserved areas of cities and rural parts of the country with less access to affordable medical care. Helping people obtain healthy food, control chronic diseases more affordably and sustainably, and deal with psychological trauma in holistic ways are things we should be doing for all patients, not just wealthy ones, so I am heartened by the great work highlighted by this group.

The most important element of changing our medical system is making and taking the time to listen to patients. Not only might the patient then be more likely to tell us the right diagnosis and treatment, but simply providing a listening ear can promote healing. Starting with teaching medical students and residents, doctors can learn that chronic diseases need not always be lifetime diagnoses and need not always steadily progress to further morbidity. This will in turn give patients the confidence to believe change is possible and that it is within their grasp. Feeling empowered as a patient helps physicians too, lifting the burden and expectation that we have the power to heal and are solely responsible for healing. That is, as we discussed at the beginning of this chapter, impossible.

Another benefit of taking more time with patients is delay and possible avoidance of judgment. A patient of mine told me that the best thing about me for himself and his wife was it felt safe to come to me with any concern, question, or symptom and not feel criticized. He said, "Both of us have had far too many doctors express contempt, anger, or displeasure if we raise a question or concern outside of that doctor's comfort zone." The only reason this is so, at least in my opinion, is because I structured my private practice to allow plenty of time for discussion. I was never required to make snap judgments on what medication to prescribe, I didn't have to limit an appointment to "one issue at a time," and I could ask questions of them in turn. I had time to find out why they asked a question I didn't understand or why they thought I might lead them to try a treatment or practice that might harm them. I had time for compassion instead of judgment. This is how most doctors I know would rather practice.

Although my practice wasn't an economic model most doctors would be happy with, it could be if the rest of the system shifted to favor high quality "slow" medicine. Practicing medicine the slow way is the only sustainable way to move forward. Focusing on allowing bodies to heal and preventing illness rather than only on intervention-based treatments will save money in the long run, while truly helping people heal and live healthier, happier lives, no matter their age. Sustainable Medicine practices strengthen doctor-patient relationships, improve quality of life for patients, and save money over time. It's up to those of us who are willing to think outside the box to support and implement these avenues to actual healing, rather than the current baseline of medical practice that is reactive and symptom-focused and better limited to emergency rooms and urgent care facilities. A good starting point is to allow Western medicine to function as emergency medicine, while shifting primary care to preventative medicine and disease reversal. It just makes practical sense.

3

HOW TO TREAT COMPLEX BEINGS SUCCESSFULLY

Every action we take in our own lives, for ourselves and for others, reverberates through the complex system we are part of, changing our health, the health of our loved ones, and the health of the planet.

When you see a person as a complex system and understand that no problem exists in a vacuum, you have the ability to see wider possibilities for healing than the average doctor or patient. The key is to keep switching your lens focus between far and close as you work through each symptom or disease constellation. Over the last century in particular, we have used technology to learn how many systems and molecules function in the body. But in narrowing medicine's focus to nutrients instead of food, whether a blood pressure of 120 or 125 is a better goal, and how much of which type of sleep-inducing medication is less likely to cause death in the long run, we've rather lost the plot. For chronic diseases and disease prevention, laser-focused thinking without whole-patient consideration can be detrimental, not just unhelpful.

In chapter two, it was clear that my patient Polly's problems were layered. Let's step back and look at her larger life picture. Having scoliosis as a younger person likely caused the wear on her knees to be uneven, which predisposed her to develop severe arthritis over many decades. Responding to an intense job she loved built up habits of pushing through stress and putting on a controlled, cheerful front, but also led to a tendency to internalize stress and push on despite pain. Years of not drinking fluids during the day to maximize active time at her job caused chronic dehydration, and perhaps even a tendency to eat more at meals, since thirst is often mistaken for hunger.

When a crisis occurred in her eighth decade in the form of a fall, her body lost the ability to compensate for the new system insults. The missed fracture in an already arthritic joint caused more pain, led to rapid worsening of her arthritis, and further destabilized her gait. Pain added to habitual stress created anxiety and elevated blood pressure that was difficult to bring down with medicines. The forced decrease in activity led to weight gain and reduced ability of her body to handle blood sugar. Dehydration, artificially reduced blood pressure when she was not in pain, and a pain medication that decreased blood flow to the kidneys all combined to hurt her kidney function.

So when Polly walked into my office for the first time, slowly and carefully using her walker, sitting precisely with her back rod-straight, and taking out her sheaf of medical notes and records from her case, she appeared to me to be a "normal" 80 year old who was moving rapidly towards the "usual" frailty of the elderly. What set her apart however, was her mental capacity and tenaciousness. I believe that her firm belief that things could be better and her willingness to try new things, combined with my faith in the body's ability to heal and willingness to keep trying, regardless of severity or age, were the key ingredients that allowed us to work together successfully. Peeling back all the layers of lifestyle habits and genetic predispositions, finding the likely causes for each of them, and then beginning the task of helping the body heal itself took some time and patience on both her part and mine.

When someone comes into an emergency room or doctor's office with a complaint that is serious or seems new, our job as physicians is to ask questions about the current problem and see if there is a way to "fix" it. We have antibiotics that work quickly, surgical procedures and trauma management to save lives within minutes or hours, and medicines like insulin and blood pressure reducers to bring various measured numerical values back into a safe range within minutes. We provide these things daily, and with these technologies there comes a feeling of control that we and patients both enjoy; in the battle against illness and death, we can wield weapons of healing that bring people back from the brink and resolve whatever serious problem has occurred.

But is this story of how medicine works true? Not as often as we wish. Sometimes the medications we choose don't work well—or at all. Sometimes surgery fails or another problem "loses the battle" for us, while we work against the first problem we thought was the most pressing. Afterwards, we might reason that the antibiotic wasn't the right one for this patient's particular bacterial type, maybe the person didn't arrive in time for surgery to save them, or after the third blood pressure medicine doesn't work, maybe we finally get a lab value back we can treat and can give a different medicine, or we replace their low magnesium and then the person stabilizes. But what is really happening?

Leonid Gavrilov, a research scientist at the Center on Aging of the National Opinion Research Center in Chicago, suggests (as discussed by Atul Gawande in his brilliant book *Being Mortal*) that "human beings fail the way all complex systems fail, gradually and randomly."[44] We are built with multiple backup systems, and backup systems for the backup systems. We have extra organs and exquisitely complex DNA repair systems. We even have what has been called "biological dark matter" (a vast improvement on the term "junk DNA"), which is flexible, adaptable, and we have no idea yet what it does—yet it makes up 95 percent of our genetic material.[45] Even more fascinating, epigenetic research has taught us that DNA gets turned on and off based on our diet, lifestyle, environmental exposures, and exercise.[46]

Complexity theory is an interdisciplinary field that studies patterns of interactions and behaviors that have many different components. Scientists working with this theory integrate hard sciences like physics and biology with humanities like sociology and economics. It is widely applied to many types of systems and is currently one of the best ways we have of modeling systems with abundant variables.[47] This theory and its modeling principles are used heavily in environmental science, and even economists are now looking at using ecological modeling techniques to better understand economic systems.[48] The human body and human decision making are areas where complexity theory has trouble, simply because of the huge number of variables. In certain instances like dealing with epidemiological data, however, this type of modeling is very helpful at teasing out which illnesses are most prevalent and what variables are consistent (or not) in those areas.

Complexity theory assumes that if we study outcomes and behaviors long enough, patterns will emerge, and we will be able to understand and even manipulate variables to influence outcomes. This is what doctors already do with patients, of course. But given how our bodies heal and become ill in ways we don't yet understand, given there are connections between mind and body we have a hard time measuring or even witnessing, and given the vast number of economic and social variables involved with human choices, it is really quite a miracle that we can help patients heal at all!

Medicine also keeps evolving, and it is to be expected that what one generation of doctors believes to be absolutely true might differ for the next generation. But these days, our medical truths seem to change year-by-year and month-by-month. We used to believe that the brain always shrinks as we age and that we can't grow new brain cells. We now know depression shrinks the brain faster than normal aging, and techniques like meditation can rebuild it.[49] We have learned that sleep allows for "rinsing" toxins out of the brain and that the brain has its own lymphatic system no one knew about until 2015.[50] [51] These new developments have huge implications for Alzheimer's disease and other neurological problems that seemed incredibly difficult to address before. Discovering such a small set of channels and finding out how sleep is even more functional than we knew suddenly shed new light on the immune system, inflammation, and toxin buildup like Alzheimer's plaques.

Cancer research is another area where science is leaping and bounding forward. It is amazingly complex these days, and now options for chemotherapy, immunotherapy, genetic therapy, focused radiation, and surgery make cancer treatments and cures more common and plausible than ever before in human history. But some of the treatments cause other cancers, some don't work well, and chemotherapy is still largely very difficult for patients' bodies to handle. Recently it was discovered that the way chemotherapy has been researched all along was missing a seemingly obvious variable: why test the drug in a 2-dimensional cell matrix petri dish when the body is 3-dimensional?[52] This simple but previously overlooked research adjustment has changed how we research the way cancers metastasize and how chemotherapy agents work. Its implications may rapidly change every ~~single~~ chemotherapy protocol now in existence, bringing back drugs that may not have worked in 2-D but might in 3, and shifting our focus away from only tumor shrinkage and growth into cell movement.

But why do both research and treatment end up so complicated and at times contradictory? Simply put, it's because the human system is so complex. Our brains are good, and computers can be better for deciphering more complex computations. However, it seems that as we get down to smaller and smaller divisions and details of how many variables there really are working in concert, we only uncover more and more information and more and more variables. Alan Watts, one of my favorite thinkers, tells it like this:

> We define (and so come to feel) the individual in the light of our narrowed "spotlight" consciousness which largely ignores the field or environment in which he is found. "Individual" is the Latin form of the Greek "atom"—that which cannot be cut or divided any further into separate parts. We cannot chop off a person's head or remove his heart without killing him. But we can kill him just as effectively by separating him from his proper environment...
>
> This implies that the only true atom is the universe—that total system of interdependent "thing-events" which can be separated from each other only in name. For the human individual is not built as a car is built. He does not come into being by assembling parts, by screwing a head on to a neck, by wiring a brain to a set of lungs, or by welding veins to a heart. Head, neck, heart, lungs, brain, veins, muscles, and glands are separate names but not separate events, and these events grow into being simultaneously and interdependently. In precisely the same way, the individual is separate from his universal environment only in name. When this is not recognized, you have been fooled by your name. Confusing names with nature, you come to believe that having a separate name makes you a separate being. This is—rather literally—to be spellbound."[53]

How does this fallacy of separation relate to medicine? Since the first mothers with sick children and the first "medicine people," the pattern of behavior in medical science has been to focus on individual variables like symptoms, then to figure out collections of symptoms, and then, pairing them with evidence (scientific or spiritual or experiential), to begin grouping symptoms with individual, identifiable diseases and with treatments that seem to work. Over time, as technical science has improved, we have found smaller and smaller biological processes that can sometimes be altered by newly created medicine molecules. Statistics regarding individual diseases are studied and sometimes environmental or cultural correlations are found. Sometimes we connect diseases with diet or lifestyle choices, and sometimes with psychological problems.

But the predominant way current doctors are trained to look at a patient is to separate the body and bodily processes from the core of the person. We dissect and we analyze and we organize. We tend to separate the person from their environment most of the time, except for asking if there is drinking or drugs involved, and perhaps if the patient is married or has children. And despite knowing that many diseases have genetic and family links, we rarely treat a whole family when one has an illness, especially a chronic one. We divide, name, and separate, and lose the forest for the trees.

History Talking: How Doctors "See" Patients

The way medical students are taught to present a patient is to see a collection of variables and tease out the "relevant" ones. A typical outpatient presentation on a patient given by a third- or fourth-year medical student sounds something like this:

This is a 49-year-old female with a history of controlled type II diabetes, here today with a sinus infection. She states she caught a cold two weeks ago and has had a fever and worsening headache since then. Other review of systems negative. She takes 500 mg of metformin twice daily and has no allergies to medications. Positive physical exam findings: she is obese, in no apparent distress, slightly elevated temperature of 99.0, blood pressure 130/80, heart rate 90. She has pain to palpation over her left maxillary sinus and shotty lymphadenopathy on her anterior left cervical chain. She has cobblestoning in the posterior larynx, but tympanic membranes are clear, lungs are clear, and no other abnormalities. Previous laboratory work up to date within two months for her diabetes. Assessment and plan: acute sinus infection, prescribe antibiotic, return to clinic if symptoms do not improve.

If the student was above average and had time, they might have asked a question about sinusitis history, and found out the woman had frequent sinus infections, at least twice a year, along with antibiotic regimens for those and other ailments up to four times a year. The student might even have looked through the previous medical record to find out what antibiotics had been given, and asked how the patient responded each time. Some might recommend a consult to a specialist, an ear, nose, and throat doctor, to make sure there wasn't something being missed that caused so many infections. An excellent student might have even asked about acid reflux symptoms, sleep apnea, then sleep quality and daily tiredness, and, if given time, about adherence to a diabetic diet. These answers might end up in the official chart note, but if the attending doctor was pressed for time, they might not change the assessment and plan right away. But maybe those would be revisited if, a week later, the patient came back if the antibiotic failed to help her symptoms.

Medical students are hopefully taught more often now that antibiotics alter the entire gut microbiota and reduce diversity there for months after the regimen is finished. They are likely taught that sleep apnea is more common in obese people and can cause high blood pressure. They might know that poor sleep is associated with weight gain. But they are rarely taught how to integrate this extra knowledge in a short outpatient visit that is scheduled to deal with one acute problem like sinus pain and fever in the usual 10 minutes allocated.

Time is definitely an issue, especially in a busy primary care practice. For this imaginary patient, her appointment scenario could look differently if her primary physician knew her well and was excellent at diagnosis. The attending would read the medical student's report, perhaps ask a few other questions of the student, then go in to examine the patient himself. He might be able to quickly ask her how her occasional reflux was doing and if she'd been sleeping. He might suggest that she take a day off of work with a note from him, get extra sleep while her children were at school, use a neti pot, drink hot liquids, and eat no dairy or meat for a couple of days, and see if her sinus pain improved. If he had a trusting relationship with her, he might even give a prescription for an antibiotic but tell her to wait a few days to fill it, since she may still have inflammation from her original virus. He might be able to convince her to see if rest and avoidance of her preference for creamy coffee and heavy foods in favor of hot tea and soups could better allow her sinuses to drain.

But this better-case scenario for a short appointment with a well-known patient still doesn't go far enough to allow the patient to stop or reverse her cycles of illness. After this appointment, if she improves with or without antibiotics, both she and her physician expect her to have a sinus infection again in the next year. They both expect her to be on metformin for the rest of her life, and at least the physician expects that she will need more medications. Every visit, he will keep checking her sugar levels and kidneys and blood pressure and add medicines as necessary to continue to stave off complications from her diabetes. He will likely mention diet and exercise, but in most cases this leads to a conversation that goes something like this (clearly I've had this conversation before in medical school!):

D: "So how is your diet going?"

P: "Great. I still love my macaroni and cheese with the kids sometimes, but most days I eat salad for lunch at work and make sure we have veggies at dinner. I never used to do that, so I think I'm doing much better. I tried switching to diet soda but I hated it, but I like sweet tea, so I figured that was better."

D: "Good start. Keep working on finding drinks that don't have sugar in them. Your numbers look stable. Just make sure to watch ~~those~~ portion sizes. If you'd like to go back to that diabetes dietician for a refresher, let me know and I'll give you a referral. What about exercise?"

P: "I run after the kids most of the day, and I'm on my feet all the time at work, so I get a lot of exercise. I might even have lost a few pounds this summer, but last weekend my brother had a birthday so that might have gone out the window!"

D: "Can you go up a flight of stairs just getting a little out of breath?"

P: "Oh yeah, we have stairs at the house. I go up and down them all day after the kids."

D: "So you don't have any shortness of breath or chest pain with exercise?"

P: "Nope, just tired from work and kids."

D: "All right then, we'll see you back in 3-4- months. You can make your appointment out front."

This is pretty decent from a Western medicine standpoint. The doctor makes sure the patient isn't having worrying symptoms that would prompt further testing. The conversation also shows that she understands the basics and is trying to comply with the recommendations for lifestyle changes that come with her diabetes diagnosis. But neither patient nor doctor expects her to do more than the minimum. Change is hard, and many patients with busy lives and other more immediate-seeming stresses are happy to hear their numbers are okay from blood work and think that means the disease process is under control and they are doing "enough." Even if this patient has seen family members suffer complications from inadequately controlled diabetes, there is often a fatalistic attitude that those things could happen to her, but it is paired with an invulnerable sense that "it might not happen to me" or "it's not happening now—I would pay more attention to my health if it were."

From the doctor's perspective, a referral to a dietician is a Hail Mary pass that he hopes makes a difference. Most doctors don't have the knowledge, the interest, or the time to discuss food with patients, much less types of exercise and sleep hygiene, especially if those weren't included in the specific reason the person came to the clinic that day. The doctor hopes that with more information and someone else encouraging her, the patient might find the motivation to change her habits. But if this patient progresses, as is usually the case, over time she will need more medications and possibly referrals to specialists for blood pressure or heart or kidney problems. If for some reason it becomes difficult to control her blood sugars, she may develop other symptoms like poor immune function and tingling pain in her feet. These sorts of things are expected and accepted with resignation by both patients and doctors. But what if there were simple ways to figure out how to reverse this trend?

A New Way to "See" a Patient

Not every appointment can be a life-changing talk about a patient's diagnoses and prognosis, but a real conversation about how their illness is affecting them, what they are doing proactively, and what might be more helpful can and should happen once or twice a year. Even for patients without a defined "Western" diagnosis, a yearly serious conversation could catch many potential problems before they become defined and entrenched. Longer appointments at more frequent intervals can also help to ensure patients actually understand their disease process and what they might be doing to slow it or accelerate it.

A conversation where the authoritarian physician says something like "You need to do this, or else" is not helpful. That rarely, if ever, works and mostly causes the patient to feel distant from and disliked by the physician. A good way to have this conversation is first to think about the person's health as a large interwoven system. There are no body parts or organ systems or emotional issues or family complications or environmental concerns that don't connect to everything else.

I can't tell you how often I've read in a history and physical, "social history: non-contributory," or "family history: non-contributory." That is never true—even in cases of adoption, emergency room visits for accidents, or pre-surgical clearance forms for a minor procedure. Maybe it can't be addressed fully then, but those things definitely contribute to how we will care for the patient and what is important to them. It might seem overwhelming both to patients and doctors to sort through all the personal habits, cultural issues, and family patterns of behavior that contribute to ill health. This is one of the reasons why the main objective of health care has been whittled down to stabilization and "management" of most chronic health problems, rather than reversal of chronic disease and healing of illness.

Of course there are counterexamples here, and drastic

measures that do have some good results. Bariatric surgery, for instance, physically curbs the amount a patient can eat and sometimes speeds up the digestion of their food so fewer calories are absorbed. I won't go into the awful side effects and short-lived benefits many patients experience, but for some, drastic procedures like that can be life saving. There are severely restrictive diets and "medical food" preparations that cause rapid weight loss, and many patients can keep some ~~of the~~ weight off while experiencing better control of blood sugars, blood pressure, and decreases in chronic inflammatory symptoms like asthma. But I hesitate to call most of those patients "healed" from their illnesses, mostly because the underlying causes of those illnesses are usually not fully addressed and the habits changed by the procedure are rarely changed for life. Since each human is a complex system, failing to address contributors like lifestyle, genetic predisposition, and microbiome dysregulation causes the body to have to compensate for those choices that tax it, and without changes in behaviors that cause the body stress, those behaviors will likely result in illness again down the line.

You might be wondering what ideas I have besides moving into someone's house, cleaning out their kitchen, ensuring they have enough financial support, taking them to buy healthy food, teaching them to cook, helping with stress management, and leading them in healthier choices, like daily exercise. While I'd be perfectly willing to do that, this is more time and energy than practicing doctors have to offer each patient, and there is no guarantee that after I left those habits would stick. I can't even make good choices for my own health 100 percent of the time, and I don't expect patients to do so without good reason and their own personal experience that it benefits them.

My Practice

In my practice, I put a lot of time into reviewing patient's medical histories, including daily routines, food, and exercise choices. It helps me see the pattern of someone's habits, preferences for certain foods, typical quantities of food, and how much time they spend sitting or working or spending time with family. When it comes time to suggest changes, knowing that much detail makes the discussion much easier and less vague.

The key thing to remember is this: complex systems are built with backups for backups for backups. We have compensating mechanisms for almost every kind of daily stressful event. If we don't sleep, we have adrenaline and cortisol to keep us moving. If we eat poorly, our gut bacteria change to species that can get more energy from our food and keep us moving. If we don't exercise, our blood pressure goes up to move our fluids and wastes to keep us detoxifying just enough to get by. If we sit for too long, our intestines work harder by retaining water and waste until we have time to relax, or stress can lead to rapid elimination, which further adds to our worries. Stress, poor nutrition, and lack of sleep cause us to store more sugar and fat for the "emergency" situation our body perceives we are in. Fatigue causes us to favor sugary foods, which in turn keep our fat cells in storage mode instead of using that food for energy. We adapt. It takes energy and causes long-term damage, but our bodies keep us alive, even when we're not able to care for them well.

Over time, all these forced compensations can lead to illness. Illness comes earlier for some of us, later for others, chronic for some of us, and in acute emergencies for others. A common trend and stereotype for "lifestyle diseases" is for abdominal fat storage to lead to inflammation with diabetes and high blood pressure as beginning diagnoses. But some patients might instead notice skin ailments or allergies, chronic intestinal discomfort, depression symptoms, or simply more frequent viral and bacterial illnesses. These, too, can be a symptom of backup systems failing to compensate well for stress.

Eastern medicine pays close attention to "stages of disease." Stages 1 through 3 rarely even cause noticeable symptoms for a patient, while stages 4 and 5 may have names for constellations of symptoms like headaches and IBS. Stage 6 is what we typically worry about in Western medicine, with serious names like diabetes and heart disease. In non-Western medical systems, prevention and catching problems early is valued much more highly than managing symptoms of a "horse already escaped out of the barn." Serious and chronic symptoms mean prevention has failed, and stage 6 diseases of the "lifestyle" type then require drastic measures, including medications, to change the behavior and health of the patient.

In Chinese, Tibetan, and Indian medicine systems, such problems cause people to be put on regimens of rigorous cleansing and exercise to create psychological change. They are given strong herbs or acupuncture as well. These systems are much better at being honest about the deadliness of the behaviors that often lead to these problems. Even if someone is predisposed by their family genes, it is taken to mean that they simply need to work harder than the average person to maintain health. Everyone has a genetic predisposition for something, so Eastern medicine's approach is to pragmatically deal with whatever cards you have been dealt conscientiously and thoroughly.

With the Western paradigm of medicine encroaching on other cultures, it may be harder now to see how much better at prevention some of these systems can be. The brilliance of modern medicines and treatments may overshadow the less miraculous ability of common sense suggestions for improving behaviors like diet and sleep. But now that Western medicine has been shown to be inadequate for prevention and reversal of chronic diseases, these older practices are becoming more popular as Western patients begin to investigate them.

Even in healthy patients with excellent genetic luck, the same sorts of stresses that cause chronic illness also eventually lead the body to break down in what we assume are "normal" results of aging. What we label "getting old" involves memory loss, arthritis, constipation, skin spots and thinness, weak hearts and lungs, along with cancers and immune system breakdown. But these effects don't happen equally to everyone, don't happen all at once, don't happen in isolation, and in many cases can be partially reversed or alleviated.

Incremental Illness Can Often Be Walked Back Incrementally

Let's step back and widen the focus briefly for some of these listed "old" diagnoses. Memory loss is worst in patients who have had sleep problems, and rapidly worsens when patients also have hearing loss, depression, or anxiety. Arthritis progresses more rapidly when muscle weakness is also present, and seems to be worst in patients with untreated structural abnormalities like scoliosis, leg length differences, and poorly compensated injuries. Constipation is worse with dehydration, lack of exercise, and with processed food diets low in whole grains and good fats. Skin breakdown is worse with dehydration and poor nutrition, and improves with proper skin care. Obviously all the major organ systems benefit from good nutrition and exercise, and many studies have been done on exercise in the elderly, proving falls can be prevented, muscle mass can be increased, and brain function can be improved.

I can't count the number of times I've heard from patients and friends the phrase "I'm just getting old" when excusing symptoms or discomfort or a new chronic diagnosis. Somehow the idea of aging and illness are so synonymous that people have become numb to most diagnoses of chronic diseases long before most of us could truthfully be considered "old." Every time someone says that, especially friends still in their thirties, I can't help but ask what they mean and why they believe it. Yes, it's true that some problems have accumulated over decades, and although they can be improved, we may not have time in this lifetime to completely reverse all damage that has happened. But no matter the problem, no matter the age of the patient, no matter if it involves a terminal illness, something can always be improved. Pain can be lessened, and suffering certainly can be. Comfort can be increased. One of the most encouraging studies I've read about aging showed that having a sense of purpose in life kept the study participants' physical bodies in better shape longer, too.[54] In the case of someone who likely has several years left, the disease process itself can be slowed or stopped, gaining the person years of healthier functioning. In cases where reversal is possible, not only can the individual regain function, but sometimes the patient will feel better in one year than they had in the past 20. This is not exaggeration. I've worked with many patients who have had excellent and unexpectedly brilliant outcomes, and I've seen other physicians do the same.

The key is to pay attention to the patient's *entire* complex system. Notice which systems are taxed the most and take the pressure off of those first, if possible. Look at what habits are the most harmful and make those the first priority when looking for small things to improve. It's easiest to think of these in terms of broad categories: sleep/rest, digestion/nutrition, elimination/lymph drainage, and exercise/metabolism. Ask what is most important to a patient during their day, what food they enjoy the most and why, and find out how they cope with stress, so you can identify better tools you can offer them.

A teacher of mine often said, "Nothing succeeds like success." The most important part of a treatment plan is to make it doable for the patient. This means being flexible, creative, and taking the time to figure out together what things to prioritize. Maybe for a patient with multiple allergies, it isn't changing their diet or getting rid of the carpet in their house, but first helping them sleep or de-stress, or eliminating fragrances in their household soaps and cleansers. If someone is firmly a "night owl," although you know it would help their metabolism to sleep differently, perhaps right now they are only amenable to exercise changes to promote weight loss. It is important to start with a simple suggestion about something they are already motivated for and aware of fully, making it more likely they will try it and succeed. Succeeding helps patients see that they *can* make changes in habit patterns, and allows deeply held assumptions to be challenged without direct confrontation.

And if, in the end, you find together that the patient is having a crisis of faith, if their job is ruining their self-esteem, or they are staying involved in relationships that are detrimental, you will likely need help in order to best help them. The same is true if their economic situation is dire, if they have traumas you are not able to help them deal with, or if the problems are simply too complicated for one person to tackle. This doesn't mean "refer and wash your hands." It means continuing to prescribe the Western drugs that buy them time, asking for help from other health care providers and social workers, and making even smaller adjustments with them that can succeed. All of which gives both of you time to work on actually healing their complex system, even if it's slow, even if it's so gradual it's hard to see changes.

The Beauty of Infinite Variables

> *The best thing about a complex system is that there are myriad angles from which to change the entire pattern.*

This means, broadly, don't give up, as a patient or a physician. We know this in some ways—many people respond to medications differently, and some patients have a harder time with routine minor surgeries than others. We are taught to adapt to different patients' needs in medical school—to a point. But the principles of adaptation and creativity apply to "lifestyle medicine" more than to any other part of medicine. And at the end of the day, there are no problems that cannot be at least palliated. Our job as physicians is to first, do no harm, and second, do what we can. There are of course time constraints, financial restraints, and noise from government and insurance and pharmaceutical companies that get in the way of being the type of doctors many of us wanted to be when we started. But we can still do much better, and we can help each other do better, too.

The rest of the chapters in this book give more concrete examples of how the individual human body is affected by things like diet, sleep, exercise, and our microbiome, and even discuss how palliative care principles can help every patient. For now, I say to both doctors and patients, start with yourself and think about how connected you are to everything around you, and how each piece of your life affects your health. Imagine your sleep pattern, the room you sleep in, and the environment of the city or town in which you live. Think of the grocery store where you purchase most of your food and the people who work there; where do the products come from and do you know any of the staff at the store? Think about your job and how you get to work, and what you like do to outside of work. Think about the past month, and remember your worst day and best day and how you handled both. Think of people you care about, how your relationships affect each other, and how they support or undermine healthy choices. Look at the wider circle of acquaintances and people you interact with on a daily basis in your community, and think of how you might affect each other.

Now remember the last time you saw a doctor or dentist or

nurse and how that interaction went. Remember the last time you paid for a haircut or clean laundry or fast food, and your interaction with the person who provided the service. Think about your news sources and how you learn. Do you view the world around you as dangerous and something to be overcome, or as friendly and helpful to you? Look at the types of personal care products and cleaning products you use on a daily or weekly basis, and think about where they come from and what the absorption of those ingredients into your lungs and skin might do. Take a quick look at your diet and exercise choices over the past few days, and evaluate how you feel physically. Is your body energetic and ready to take on your next task? Do you wake up refreshed and excited about your day?

You can see that there are hundreds and thousands of small interactions every day with other people, with food, with the air you breathe, and with your own thoughts. You can begin to imagine the web you are part of, and see that every single, tiny decision affects something else. Your body itself is a web of simultaneous interactions within your larger community-sized web, within the planetary web we depend on to live. Each decision you make, even how you think, affects every system at once. Nothing exists in isolation. I suggest we first learn about the variables in our individual lives, then find out how to take better care of ourselves, and allow those positive actions to extend out from us. Even if you are a physician or health care practitioner reading this and want to focus on patients primarily, it is still true that taking care of yourself first is necessary to have the energy to help others. Every action we take for ourselves and for others in our lives reverberates through the complex system we are part of, changing our health, the health of our loved ones, and the health of the planet.

4

SLEEP: ON BEING PHOTOPERIODIC MAMMALS

Chronobiology

Biological time, or chronobiology, is one of my favorite concepts in science. The idea that biological processes in living organisms are affected by the cycles of light and dark and the turning of the moon and the earth is something that indigenous societies seem to have always known and absorbed into their cultures. Over the last few centuries though, more "civilized" or "developed" societies have been able to ignore the idea of biological rhythms in progressively oppositional ways. We've developed lights that keep us working and playing all night and jobs that ask us to work second or third shifts. Most people who need to be at work at a set time require alarm clocks because of chronic exhaustion. Our computer and phone screens have bright lights that make it easy to read, watch videos, and perform complicated artistic feats, but the short wave light they emit confuses our natural sleep-wake cycles.[55]

There are numerous studies on how poor sleep affects our health, from diabetes to Alzheimer's to depression and risk for suicide.[56] [57] [58] [59] [60] [61] [62] [63] [64] [65] There are also plentiful studies on how improvements in sleep help repair damage to our bodies, especially regarding aging and mental health.[66] [67] [68] In two very recent studies, scientists found that during the part of sleep called REM sleep (rapid eye movement, or deep dreaming sleep), toxins are "rinsed" out of the brain,[69] [70] likely via the newly discovered lymphatic system in the central nervous system that astonished anatomists and neuroscientists.[71] [72] These new findings are completely changing how we think about and treat many illnesses involving the nervous system, like Alzheimer's, meningitis, and multiple sclerosis. Sleep is a vital healing topic I learned the most about long after medical school.

Let me tell you about a patient of mine with type 1 diabetes, whom I'll call Jordan (and I'm altering some details to keep his real information private). Jordan had first been diagnosed as a thirty year old, and although he had been vigilant and done his best with medications and diet recommendations, by the time he was nearing sixty, he had several complications affecting his circulation and metabolism. He was worried about his memory and frequently felt frustrated, which was affecting his relationship with his spouse. Even though his illness was becoming increasingly difficult to deal with, he was an expert at counting carbohydrates and made sure to give himself exactly the right amount of insulin for everything he ate.

Before I met Jordan, most doctors throughout his life had focused strictly on food and medication to keep his blood sugar numbers in check. I was apparently the first doctor who had ever asked about his sleep habits. It turned out he was going to sleep at 2 a.m., having a snack before bed, and taking a small amount of insulin at that time. Around 5 a.m. many mornings, he would awaken shaking and sweating, his heart racing, and with dangerously low blood sugar. He would then drink orange juice to raise his blood sugar in order to avoid having a more serious complication requiring a visit to the hospital. A bit later, before lunch, his blood sugar would be very high and would require extra insulin, even before he accounted for his food. His lab results were very good despite these episodes, so his insulin regimen hadn't been changed in some time. He was feeling sick, exhausted, and had a hard time answering questions in my office due to his high level of frustration.

It was clear to me what was happening, mostly due to the Ayurvedic training I had just completed. Around 10 p.m., since he didn't go to sleep at a time his body naturally would want to, he likely had extra adrenaline and cortisol circulating, keeping him alert late into the night, which would also make his blood sugar drop, causing the craving for a carbohydrate snack. He'd eat, take his insulin to compensate, and then finally feel exhausted enough to sleep. A few hours later, the natural early morning release of cortisol and adrenaline would try to raise his blood sugar levels in preparation for waking in the morning, but the insulin would keep it artificially low. This would precipitate an emergency his body had to compensate for, which produced his symptoms. This almost daily cycle made him even more exhausted, sleeping long into the afternoon, while his hormones and metabolism worked overtime just to keep him alive.

So we decided to first change his sleep routine, to include both more sleep earlier at night and exposure to early morning sunlight. I warned that it might be hard to change his sleep habits, since he'd been a night owl for so long. I suggested he see what he could do, call me with questions, and return to see me in a month. Two weeks later he appeared in my office, smiling. He asked me to check his lab work, but it was too soon to be of any use, so I asked him, "Why?" He said that after two weeks of going to bed earlier he hadn't had ONE low blood sugar episode and had reduced his daily insulin dose on his own by several units. I was really proud of him, but quite shocked it had worked so quickly. Since he felt better and was interested, we adjusted a few other minor things in his diet and routine and scheduled him to return in a month.

When he returned for another checkup, his daily blood sugars had improved so much that his daily doses of longer-acting insulin needed to be lowered substantially. He felt his memory had improved, he had more energy, and he was getting much more done with his work and hobbies than he had in years. Best of all, he had been in such a better frame of mind that his relationship was less strained, to both partners' relief.

The only thing we'd really done was to make sure he aimed to go to sleep around 10 p.m. He seemed to need less sleep this way as well, was more productive during the day, needed less medication, and was feeling better psychologically than he had in a long time. We were all amazed by his results, but I think I was most of all. Nothing during medical school or residency had taught me the huge effect sleep could have on a patient's health and quality of life—even in someone at a late stage of chronic illness like Jordan. I started to realize what an even larger difference this might have made in his health had he been sleeping at a more reasonable time through the years. It astounded me I wasn't taught to prioritize the sleep patterns that ancient science emphasized and even treated early illness with. Although usually less dramatic, this concept is true for many patients with many different types of illnesses and symptoms.

Your Built-in Alarm Clock

How the human internal clock works is both simple and complex. The simple part is that daily light signals our brain, which then tells our body's systems when to do which function, and this all changes monthly and seasonally. The complicated part is, like absolutely everything in the human body, we're not exactly sure how every part of the sleep cycle works. We also have very little detailed knowledge about all the ways our systems are affected by the sleep cycle, especially what happens when it is not regular.

Feedback from our body's systems back and forth to our brains involves so many variables, we have only discovered about a tenth of them, which is a generous estimate in my opinion. We know for sure though, when sleep is excellent, people live longer, happier, healthier lives, with less cancer and symptoms of aging.

Our pineal gland gets light information second-hand from our eyes through the superchiasmatic nucleus (SCN), which relays the message that it's daytime through the sympathetic nervous system to our pineal gland. The SCN fires most rapidly at noon and slowest at night, and has melatonin receptors itself, which provide feedback and slow its firing rate. The science is clear on this part, since injury or a problem at the SCN results in severe circadian rhythm disorders.

To understand this better, we can start by examining our clock's basic mechanism. The pineal gland, tiny and pine-cone-shaped, produces the hormone melatonin, which affects every organ system in the body and is the primary regulator of our daily sleep-wake cycles, usually referred to as the circadian rhythm. The pineal sits right between our brain hemispheres, between the two halves of the thalamus, surrounded by cerebrospinal fluid. In some reptiles and amphibians, and in mammals' evolutionary histories, the same type of gland is triggered directly by light, which means the sun directly controls their circadian rhythms, as well as seasonal and yearly rhythms for body functions like reproduction. It has had a rather mystical reputation for thousands of years, and is sometimes referred to as the "third eye."

The pineal is like the adrenal glands in that it gets information about light as well as about how the whole system is doing from the sympathetic nervous system, which it then relays via hormone messengers to the rest of the body almost instantly. Many of the pineal gland's messages go straight to the pituitary gland. The pituitary also gets messages from the hypothalamus via hormones and electric signals, and combined with information from the pineal gland, regulates growth, thyroid and adrenal function, kidney function, and reproductive hormones. The amount and timing of melatonin (and likely other messengers we haven't discovered yet) helps regulate most other hormones and systemic body functions, including sleep-wake cycles, body temperature, blood pressure, menopause and puberty, blood sugar and fat storage, aging, and immune function.[73] [74] [75] The timing and length of the peak of melatonin secretion is correlated with mood and anxiety, and with quality of life.[76] If the pineal gland is damaged, its functions don't normalize if melatonin is replaced, so there are likely other ways the pineal works—we just aren't aware of them yet.

After so many decades of artificial light and new technology interfering with our sleep-wake cycles (during which time most research on melatonin has been done), we aren't sure exactly how much humans are still affected by day length, seasons, and lunar cycles. We also don't know how much melatonin is linked to those types of periodicity, but it is true that daily and monthly cycles and melatonin affect all our systems including individual cells, metabolic activity, and immunity. It is also clear that when humans don't have steady routines connected with planetary rhythms (like sleeping, eating, and elimination), we are less resilient and our health is poorer.

Connecting with our cycles and body rhythms can help keep us alert to changes and more sensitive to when we might need more rest or rejuvenation. Best of all, using light exposure to help regulate cycles may lead to more effective treatment plans for issues like infertility and premenstrual depression.[77] [78] One of my favorite (if not yet replicated) studies showed that women's cycles set themselves on a "normal" 29-day pattern when the women were given a dim light in their bedrooms simulating a full moon during the three days of their ovulatory phase.[79]

In general, for anyone with disordered sleep, the simplest and fastest way to correct the problem is to go camping for a few days without artificial light.[80] [81] The fact that humans have seasonal affective disorder at all, and that SAD is helped by light therapy, means that despite our attempts to get around the natural cycle of time, we are still photoperiodic animals. Several factors make extremely precise seasonal and daily variation in melatonin secretion possible. However, the complexity, sensitivity, and multiple feedback loops in the system mean that the system can be derailed, and more easily derailed if the main trigger of daily light variation is uncoupled from natural planetary cycles.

The following reviews the four biggest pieces of this system that have been studied the most, and gives clear examples of ways this system can be nudged out of equilibrium.

Science Break ☺

1. The pineal gland's production of melatonin is tightly controlled by several factors, including neurotransmitters and neuropeptides. Tiny deviations are noticed and amplified in a system this finely tuned, so stress-induced chronic high concentrations of epinephrine (adrenaline) and norepinephrine can strongly affect the pineal gland, and therefore sleep and other body processes.

2. Melatonin is made from serotonin, levels of which are affected by (and affect) depression and anxiety. Our gut bacteria produce most of the serotonin in the body, so psychiatric issues as well as dietary and intestinal problems affect the melatonin system and vice versa.

3. The third main thing to know is that melatonin is also produced *outside* of the pineal gland, and receptors are found nearly everywhere in the body.[82] [83] [84] [85] [86] [87] Melatonin is produced in bone marrow, immune cells, and epithelial (skin and gut lining) cells. Levels of melatonin in the intestine change with food intake and intestinal production. Receptors that respond to melatonin are found in the retina, in neurons, arteries, cancer cells, and

in the reproductive, digestive, and metabolic systems. Melatonin helps blood vessels relax, protects the heart, and boosts immune response. Variations in lifestyle, diet, illness, and medications all affect production of and response to melatonin.

4. Lastly, one of melatonin's most important functions is as an antioxidant. Oxidation and inflammation, along with genetic predisposition and epigenetic factors, are thought to lead to worsening of diseases like Alzheimer's, Parkinson's, Huntington's, ALS, epilepsy, and strokes.[88] The amount of calcification in the pineal gland, and the smaller volume of working gland, is worse in Alzheimer's patients, which might be part of what speeds up the disease process.[89]

With all this intricate feedback, it isn't just light exposure, but also stress, how long you sleep and when, exercise, diet, drugs, and other environmental and behavioral factors that affect our pineal gland's function, and with it the rest of the entire body. It wouldn't surprise me if poor sleep will be found to be strongly associated with the causes of early puberty, more prevalent menopause symptoms, neurodegenerative diseases, and psychiatric illnesses.

So far, research has mostly focused on finding a way to use melatonin as a supplement. If it worked, it would theoretically help correct problems that seem to be correlated with low melatonin levels, or even as a treatment for confusing multi-variable problems such as irritable bowel syndrome. But researchers have tried supplemental melatonin for a variety of ailments from breast cancer to menopause with ambiguous results. Supplements of melatonin seem to have a mild effect on sleep disturbances and menopausal symptoms in certain cases, but careful timing of dosing is required. In breast cancer, prostate cancer, and heart disease, melatonin levels are lower than average, and supplements could lengthen survival very slightly. For metabolic problems like insulin resistance and weight management, melatonin may be helpful in the future, but research is still inconclusive. In a study on the antioxidant properties of melatonin in neurodegenerative diseases, the authors' conclusion was that more studies are needed to recommend melatonin's use.[90]

Since this is a complex system, many of these seem a bit like the "chicken or egg" scenarios. An example might go something like this: someone predisposed to Alzheimer's disease, who has a stressful early and/or mid-life and has slept less than needed over the years, has a tendency for their pineal gland to calcify. This may be accelerated by poor sleep. Then the person happens to develop cataracts, which decrease the amount of light getting to their retinas and therefore decreases pineal function. Then, environmental influences trigger more epigenetic factors that worsen the person's sleep along with digestion and waste elimination, all of which may worsen the calcification of the pineal gland. This means the typical Western idea to "just supplement melatonin" might not be of much help, and certainly not without other (and earlier) interventions.

Melatonin affects so many systems that taking a supplement and trying to adjust the dose will affect systems across the entire body and may have unpleasant side effects and drug interactions. A quick Google search turns up side effects like nausea, headaches, dizziness, abdominal cramps, and low blood pressure. If you take medications to thin your blood, lower blood sugar, prevent seizures, or if you use birth control, melatonin can affect how those and other medicines work. Because of its complex systemic effects, melatonin is one of those supplements that is easy to take too much of, and difficult to know what dose will be effective and for whom. In contrast, improving patients' levels of melatonin with improved sleep has only positive effects, with the added benefits of internal feedback and fine-tuning that cannot be replicated with any pill. Teaching meditation to patients can also improve melatonin levels, as meditation has the effect of adjusting serotonin and norepinephrine levels, which may explain some of the mechanisms by which meditation causes so many health benefits.[91] [92]

In patients with seasonal affective disorder, phototherapy relieved their symptoms but didn't always adjust their melatonin levels, and melatonin supplements didn't work at all.[93] I wonder, in many of these cases, why not focus on doing studies where sleep itself is corrected with phototherapy and behavioral therapy, since we know sleep correction helps, and then see if the inner pharmacy's melatonin and other molecules are more effective at helping to heal SAD and other disorders? Why not do more studies on exercise and meditation, since those at least work marginally better than placebo, often better than drugs, and build brain volume even in the very old? [94] [95] [96] [97] [98] [99] [100] [101] [102] [103] [104]

From what I have seen, the primary sleep problem humans seem to have is a pervasive cultural misunderstanding of how our body keeps its healthy equilibrium. With the help of technology, many of us have become so separate from the natural cycles of our planet's day, month, and year, that our bodies' natural responses to these things seem irritating. Many of us treat sleep as an inconvenience, a waste of time, an unwanted intermission in the forward march of our progress in school, work, relationships, and leisure time. Medications to keep us awake and to help us sleep seem normal, despite the facts that these medications are associated with earlier death, injuries, and poor brain function.[105] [106] [107]

In hospitals, the places where our sickest friends and family are expected to heal, patients are awakened many times throughout the night to document vital signs and check treatment trajectory.[108] [109] Doctors make rounds before dawn to ensure they see everyone. Care is not coordinated for patient rest, but for technician and nurse convenience, especially when hospitals are chronically understaffed and patients are sicker. Our protocols and work pressure on hospital staff disregard that sleep is absolutely required for healing. Every parent knows this, and we apply it liberally to our children. We even sometimes apply it to adults who are "ill enough" to fall asleep despite their intentions to remain awake and working. But for some reason, our cultural appreciation for 24-hour technology and documentation trumps this obvious knowledge, even in medicine where healing is our primary concern.

When I was between two and three years old, I needed to be hospitalized briefly for dehydration caused by a gastrointestinal virus. After less than a day in the hospital, my mother took me home "against medical advice" because not only was I checked on by a conscientious nurse every two hours, I also shared my room with a crying baby and hadn't been able to nap at all much less sleep during that one night, even after I wasn't actively sick. After my mother brought me home, I slept for 14 straight hours. I still clearly remember waking up at a strange time, after bedtime certainly, feeling groggy and confused. I remember crawling quietly out to find my mother in the living room, thinking I might be in trouble for being awake when it was dark outside. Otherwise I felt fine, was ready to eat, and was my cheerful self again, if a little jet-lagged, after that restorative sleep. I'm sure most parents can share similar experiences, but for some reason we stop applying this simple wisdom to ourselves after childhood.

The point is that sleep is the foundation for allowing the body to heal itself, borne out by piles of research, but sleep improvement is **not** emphasized in medical school. As students and physicians in particular, we spend our training years making our bodies compensate dramatically for lack of sleep, likely contributing to the high rates of depression and anxiety experienced by medical students and physicians.[110] How can anyone have enough energy to meet challenges in their everyday life, much less handle the stress of life and death decisions in a hospital situation if they are exhausted? Many of our patients have the same issues, and since we know poor sleep contributes to everything from weight gain to Alzheimer's, it seems we are in need of a new way of teaching how sleep heals us and how to implement changes with individual patients.

In Eastern medical traditions like Ayurveda, the required timing for sleep is simple and easy to understand. The basic optimal sleep time is from 10 p.m. to 6 a.m. There is leeway an hour back and forth on both sides to accommodate individual variations in constitution, work, culture, and preference. Before going to sleep, it is recommended that people turn off lights (and screens of all kinds), listen to relaxing music, have a warm bath or massage with warm oils, converse with loved ones, and have a warm, non-alcoholic drink to calm digestion. Interestingly, the protocols in studies for helping people sleep better sound exactly like these ancient recommendations.[111] [112] Protocols like this help the body heal itself and are proven to improve sleep in hospitals. These interventions also decrease sedative use, which saves lives, brain function, and prevents injury.[113]

Teenagers, Jet Lag, and Sleeping In

So much of our brain function is reorganized and optimized during sleep. While we sleep, our brain basically works on "filing" what has happened during our day. It takes new information and decides whether to put it in the memory banks or delete it, and our dreams seem to "let off steam" from our consciousness during the heaviest working time of our unconscious brains. In more scientific terms, the brain clears out toxins, repairs damage, and rebuilds itself. During REM sleep, our brains are incredibly active, including parts that are quiet during waking hours.[114]

These functions explain why eight to nine hours of sleep are required for teenagers to properly process new information learned in order to be able to retrieve it and apply it the next day on a test. Studies on university students show similar results, with students who get adequate sleep (7 or more hours) doing better on exams.

But simply staying in bed the requisite average number of hours per week doesn't seem to make it certain that we feel rested. Catching up on weekends helps but only goes so far. Though we know that REM cycles occur in 90-minute sessions, long naps can leave us feeling almost ill rather than refreshed. So there must be something in the timing we haven't yet fully taken advantage of.

We need to redefine how we think about rest as it relates to our internal self-healing mechanisms, and not just because it is clearly needed in medicine in order for students and physicians to "prescribe" it. More importantly, redefining rest in this way connects us to our home and the natural cycles we have grown antagonistic towards, but which are vital to our well-being. Sleep, rest, stress reduction, and recovery are all human requirements. Lack of sleep causes a cascade of events signifying the brain is behind on detoxifying itself, it hasn't "filed" information correctly, and the entire body is overdue on repairing and regenerating damaged cells and systems. Even irregular sleep acts similarly to jet lag on the body, so irregular sleep on a daily basis takes a huge toll on the feedback mechanisms that are so intricately monitored and responded to by all the body's systems.[115] If we would pay attention and work to combat inadequate sleep like we do drunk driving, we would save lives from automobile and other kinds of accidents with heavy machinery, in addition to the health benefits we already talked about.[116]

So, What to Do?

For most of us, we know we feel better when we get enough sleep—but what is enough, and does when we get that sleep matter? Napping for 10-20 minutes has gotten attention lately as a way to help maintain alertness and productivity during the workday, but is that the best way to deal with fatigue? And what about people who are genetically predisposed to be "night owls?"

The best way to stop forcing your body to waste energy compensating for the added stress of an irregular schedule is to find a schedule that works for you and stick to it. To determine what regimen is best for you, we can look at what "optimal" is. Each individual will need different amounts and types of sleep and rest at different times of life, but the basic requirements are easy to modify for optimum health benefits.

Optimal sleep looks something like this (and please realize very few people have this experience, so if you do, cheers! If not, it's something to work toward): you awaken refreshed without an alarm clock sometime within an hour of sunrise, and feel energetic during the day without requiring a nap (but perhaps you experience times of lowered activity level and episodes of meditation and rest and exercise); you have dinner within an hour of sunset; you wind down and turn off screens at or before 8 p.m.; and you are asleep within an hour of 9:45 p.m., and do not awaken with insomnia during the night.

Optimal rest and stress reduction may include formal meditation practices, or any regular activities that are regenerative for the individual, as diverse as knitting, gardening, art, music, surfing, or even simple walking. One thing necessary for optimum benefit in active practices (especially for decreasing symptoms of anxiety and stress) is being in nature.[117] [118] [119] Walking on a treadmill in a gym or in a mall may increase anxiety, while just five minutes walking in nature improves mood and self-esteem.

Optimal recovery is extremely important not just for actual recovery from illness, but also for prevention of illness. When a patient is ill enough to come to the doctor's office, it's easy to tell them to rest, and there is little resistance at that point if they've already taken time off work. On the other hand, after a stressful event, a minor illness, or week at work, going all out with weekend activities and staying up late will add to the body's need to compensate to keep itself going, increasing the risk of short-term illness as well as long-term health problems.

If you have parented children, been in an intense school situation, served in the military, worked nights or emergency services, been jet lagged, or spent time in a hospital yourself, you understand how terrible it feels to have irregular sleep. You may also recall how much more likely it is to catch a cold or flu right as you think you might be coming out from under a stressful situation. It makes sense, though, given that after peak stress the "high-alert" goes down and the immune cells and stress hormones back off, making it more likely that your immune system will miss or be unable to fight off intruders. You may also recall that it is more likely that the cold will become bronchitis or a sinus infection, or that you are more likely to injure yourself while being a "weekend warrior," if your body is already at its limit of compensation.

Like we discussed in the last chapter, the causes of illness are many times simply the body's backups and reserves failing, or simply having too many negative inputs at once. Chronic illness and severe illnesses rarely happen in isolation, but rather are often the result of long-term stress on the body's multiple self-healing processes. We can encourage patients and ourselves to prevent illness and stave off long-term problems by designing a sleep and rest routine that keeps the immune system healthy and ready for action. We can encourage and practice self-knowledge about what makes us feel best, especially if we haven't felt well in a long time. We can also be vigilant about understanding how stress affects each of us individually, taking extra good care of ourselves during stressful times, and not forcing the body to cope with continued denial of its connection to the planet's circadian cycle.

If you've had poor sleep for a long time, please don't expect a pill to fix the underlying problem. Medications commonly given for sleep problems can be addictive and tolerance is built very quickly. A few even change normal sleep structure, allowing the body to be still and restful (which can be necessary during a short-term stressful situation), but the brain activity normally associated with sleep is altered, not allowing for routine detoxification and memory processing. Some of the most popular sleep drugs (benzodiazepines) simply induce anesthesia-like sedation rather than healthy, restorative sleep. Many sleep aid drugs affect mood, memory, and some even cause hallucinations. Worse, much more severe insomnia than was the initial reason for the prescription can be a rebound effect for a long period after the drug is stopped.

None of these medicines are meant to be taken for more than a night or two at a time, regardless of marketing claims, and research shows that taking even as few as 18 a year increases risk of death significantly.[120] Some of that may be due to whatever underlying issues caused the imbalance to begin with, but the studies are quite clear: if you take sleeping pills—even just Benadryl—you have a higher risk of death than if you don't.

Assess and Adjust your Sleep Routine

First take stock of your current routine. Find what obstacles to sleep are present in your lifestyle, family, sleeping room, and area you live in, such as noises, lights, or interruptions. Start with the most easily modifiable items and change those first. For those of you who have trouble staying asleep, sometimes a small intervention such as avoiding water an hour before bed or having a small healthy snack can help. Many tools exist that can be useful in building a sleep routine that works for you. There are apps and machines which generate white noise, humidifiers for dry sinuses and allergy sufferers, simple fans for noise or coolness (the ideal human sleep temperature is around 64 degrees), blackened window shades, phototherapy lamps to assist waking up, and mattress pads and pillows to help with pain and injury accommodation.

For those with difficulty finding time to sleep, knowing that it would help productivity, mood, energy, and general defense against illness might motivate you to try an experiment. Take some time off from a social schedule, and find a partner or friend to help with obligations and children for a short time. For the first week, go to bed around 9:30 p.m., making sure the pre-bed routine is restful and without screens. Many of us feel sleepy around 8 p.m., so instead of fighting the tiredness, give in and get ready for bed, finding a relaxing activity to do until 9 or so. Allow yourself to stay in bed, and then sleep as long as needed to catch up, again enlisting a friend or partner to help with morning obligations if needed. Trying this on a weekend or vacation is helpful, obviously, and going camping without artificial light is ideal. A few of my patients who have tried this slept up to 15 hours the first day they followed the routine and allowed themselves to relax enough to sleep.

What this experiment is good for, especially if you can't normally allow yourself days at a time to sleep in, is to see how long you need to feel refreshed. This is your marker. At first it will be longer, but after three to four days, sleep necessity usually levels off, and you may start feeling better rested. If it has been years since you were free to sleep as much as you needed, this will be a new feeling and it might require some time to fully catch up and feel healthy with your sleep patterns. But this short experiment will give you a guideline for the next phase, fitting your new knowledge into your existing life schedule.

Take the number of hours of sleep you've found makes you feel best and fit them as best you can around the 10 p.m. to 6 a.m. format, depending on your work schedule and family. This still might prove difficult, since frequent awakenings with issues like anxiety, needing to urinate at night, or a partner with sleep issues can be additional obstacles to good sleep, but making sure all other variables are taken care of first is a helpful start. Most people find they need around 7–8 hours of sleep in approximately 90-minute increments to allow for REM cycle optimization. Depending on how much light you can see in the morning and how long it takes for your pineal gland to improve its function, you will likely need to adjust your bedtime and rising time over the first few months to fit your needs.

It's best to get up earlier rather than later in order to catch the morning sun and get some brief exercise. Many parents find that extra time in the morning before children awaken is the most productive personal part of their day, if they can get to sleep early enough at night to make it worthwhile. If your nighttime sleep is not enough and can't be lengthened, napping and weekend catching up become necessary. In the middle of a workday, 20 minutes seems to be optimal for refreshing brain function and improving alertness and performance. A meditation session for that length of time has similar benefits, and even a non-sleep rest or brief walk may work well for you.

If time is available and you are truly sleep deprived, a 90-minute REM cycle may be needed, but be careful to set an alarm. With 90-minute naps, be aware that you still may have some grogginess after waking, although this may be less likely if the nap is taken in the morning. On weekends, for the truly exhausted, sleeping longer can help, but it is best if you can also go to bed early or on time, near 10 p.m., and then sleep as long as needed. Making an effort to take a walk in the morning light to help your melatonin levels normalize.

As you tune in more closely to your body's sleep needs, you might notice a tendency to want more sleep in the winter and less in the summer. This is actually very normal, and it's best to go with the sun as long as you're still getting enough total sleep hours. Living in Alaska or similar places very far south or north definitely necessitates blackout shades and phototherapy lights, and possibly a stricter schedule to maintain sleep health. Your basic evaluation can rely on how much energy you have during the day and whether you need an alarm clock in the morning.

It *is* possible to get too much sleep. For instance, in patients with depression, staying in bed an extra hour or more can cause worsening symptoms. I have seen this many times in my practice.

My hypothesis is that it may have to do with melatonin timing. By throwing off a sleep routine either in the morning or at night, the "jet-lag" phenomenon occurs, which causes fatigue and reluctance to exercise or maintain a routine in general. In susceptible individuals, particularly with depression, this can seriously set back a treatment program.

Exercise can help with sleep as well, toning the sympathetic nervous system to be able to shut itself off when sleep is needed. At this stage, since dealing with sleep is primary, the best time to exercise is when you can find time, and the best exercise type is one you enjoy and can continue doing! Joking aside, exercising in the morning, particularly just after sunrise, is a great way to both enliven your system for the day and help your pineal gland obtain accurate information to help you sleep better at night. Chapter 8 covers particular exercise types and has more specific recommendations. For ideal sleep, simply having a routine, even a small one that involves daytime nature walks, is best.

Now I need to make a point here to differentiate between types of sleep disorders. Some patients have issues that directly affect sleep, which need to be treated first. Examples of this type of disorder would be sleep apnea, restless leg syndrome, sleepwalking, narcolepsy, and many others. There are also people with such serious sleep difficulties they feel they are awake most of the night. What I've said above may not work for you if you are one of these people, although my suggestions are safe to try. I want to reassure you that if they don't work, there are other ways to try to improve sleep, some of which are a bit counterintuitive.

My favorite of these methods is implemented at an insomnia clinic in London, run by a psychiatrist named Hugh Selsick who specializes in serious sleep problems. His team gives patients very strict guidelines for sleep: they keep the wake-up time rigidly the same, use a minimum sleep time to improve sleep efficiency, and don't allow anyone near the bedroom unless it's for sleep (or sex)—not even to change clothes. The results? Eighty percent of patients report significant improvement and 50 percent report being cured. So, research is ongoing and it looks very promising for patients with the most severe insomnia.[121]

Summary

The first step to helping your body heal is tuning in to your circadian rhythm. We are intimately connected to the planet, the sun, and the moon. Our complex system is connected to the cycles caused by the celestial wanderings of these bodies. Optimum function of our entire endocrine system is dependent on whether we pay attention and follow the rhythm of the environment that surrounds us. The importance of this cannot be overstated. Our bodies are able to compensate for a very long time, and staying up late or being stressed for years at a time seems difficult but not impossible when we are teenagers or in our 20s. But long-term consequences of forcing our body systems to compensate take their toll, affecting our genes, metabolisms, and brains. Insufficient sleep and circadian rhythm disruption are linked to heart disease, high blood pressure, stroke, diabetes, obesity, depression, and poor brain function, not to mention increases in accidents, decrease in sex drive, and faster aging. Paying close attention to and working *with* instead of *against* our internal biological clocks can start to reverse some of these issues. If started early and used preventatively, these principles may help put off chronic illnesses even in the genetically susceptible, and sometimes entirely.

As physicians, helping patients correct circadian dysfunction is the first and most important step in helping to begin true healing. As patients ourselves, correcting our poor sleep habits will go a long way to help us help others. Sleep should always be our first "weapon" against colds and flus, but also depression and chronic illness. At the onset of a cold, make sure to first get extra sleep. When stress levels rise at home or work, make sure your circadian rhythm is on track. When your body is expending energy for illness or any other reason, make sure it doesn't have to also compensate for lack of sleep. And if some of the issues arising are preventing you from sleeping, you'll know what to do: return to your sleep routine as soon as you can to recover. If sleep problems are persistent and tricky, cognitive behavioral therapy (CBT) is a first-line treatment, and many practitioners around the country do excellent work treating insomnia with CBT.

5

WHAT SHOULD WE EAT?

One particularly happy memory I have is from when I was five years old, during one of our regular visits to my grandparents' house. My grandmother would take a piece of wonder bread, spread it with "oleo" (what she called margarine), and pile it high with store-brand peach preserves, then feed it to me by hand. My mother expressed irritation that I was being "spoiled" by the unnecessary hand-feeding, but no one was bothered by the thought that there was too much sugar in the preserves which might tax my liver and pancreas. No one thought the white bread was so devoid of nutrients to make it essentially sugar and air. And no one worried that the hydrogenated vegetable oil in the fake butter would start to clog my arteries. But all these things were true, and over time, choices like these based on faulty information and marketing lead to the chronic diseases so prevalent these days.

Foods we associate with love and comfort (like cake, hot dogs, white bread, fried foods, macaroni and cheese) are overwhelmingly high in simple carbohydrates and unhealthy fats and comparatively low in nutritional value. Most of these products actually need more sugar, salt, and fat than in a normal recipe in order to counteract the bitterness of ultra-processed grains. Soda, macaroni and cheese, canned soups, and packaged cookies all remind me positively of my childhood. The strange thing is that any time in the last 15 years I've tried one of my childhood favorites, my taste buds are bombarded with either too much salt or sugar, or both, and often a strange oily aftertaste. The memories, obviously, are much better for me than the actual foods.

I don't think anyone at this point would argue that cola or white bread is "good" for you. But our food preferences do take a long time to shift, and the big companies in the food industry are very good at producing and marketing low-nutrition, highly processed foods that the majority of Americans (and those increasingly eating Western diets across the world) purchase regularly. Some people with lucky genetics can avoid heart disease or diabetes for longer than others, but these days children as young as two have significant artery plaques,[122] [123] and additional risk factors like smoking and obesity cause much larger and extensive artery calcification. In a 2008 study of children with heart problems, 75 percent of the children (the average age was thirteen, and 57 percent were obese) had arteries that looked like those of adults near the age of forty-five.[124] And the rates of diabetes are increasing all over the world, as people adopt "Western diets" and activity levels decrease.[125]

These types of studies mean there is no time to lose to take care of our collective health. A diet that allows the body to heal, to build healthy tissue, and to recover quickly from illness or trauma is the same type of diet that will prevent illness and help start to reverse chronic diseases. Broadly, this means more whole foods in general, less meat, and much less processed food. It might also mean that periods of fasting would be beneficial[126] [127] (for an in-depth discussion about fasting, see appendix 3) and that some foods are off-limits for certain people with particular sensitivities.[128] How do we decide what's best to eat and when, and what criteria do we use?

Introducing our Microbiomes

The health of the microbes in our gut makes a huge difference in how much nutrition we obtain from what we eat. No matter how high in nutrition our food choices may be, if we can't digest well, it doesn't matter how good the food is. One of the clearest examples of digestive health being crucial to nutrition absorption is phytochemicals. Many fruits and vegetables that are marketed as "superfoods" are labeled as such because of their high content of phytochemicals. These are compounds from plants that are anti-cancer, anti-inflammatory, and immunomodulatory (modifying and training the immune system to be more efficient and less over-reactive). The kicker is that since humans can't actually digest these compounds, we cannot benefit from them unless our gut bacteria are working well.

Our intestinal tracts have 3–5 *pounds* of bacteria that are *required* for us to be able to obtain certain vitamins and make certain hormones and neurotransmitters from our food.[129] Vitamin K2, for instance, which is essential for blood clotting and healing, is only made via intestinal bacteria. Vitamin D is made in the skin first, but has to go through the liver and kidneys to become functional. It works in the intestines, regulating calcium absorption and modulating inflammation.[130] Vitamin D deficiency is correlated with all sorts of health issues, but its direct interaction with gut bacteria is also important in regulating our body's immune responses, in addition to helping us absorb calcium from our food.[131] Other dietary components like the ratio of omega-6 and omega-3 fatty acids also interact with our gut bacteria and affect our immune system and ability to regulate inflammation.[132]

We might understand that stress affects our microbiome, but we're finding out that intestinal bacteria actually send more information *to* our brains and immune system than the other way around.[133] [134] [135] [136] I'll go farther into how we can keep our microbial friends happy in the next chapter, but for now just keep them in mind when making food choices, since their survival and function depends on our ingestion of highly nutritious pre- and pro-biotic foods.

Food Diaries: Information Gathering

Doctors often tell patients to "do better with your diet" or "eat healthier." This isn't just unhelpful, it is quite assumption-filled. It *assumes* that what patients are eating is unhealthy. Secondly, it assumes patients know what to do to change their diet to a "healthier" set of foods. While sometimes people do know how they can improve their diet, it's also usually true that people are already making the best use they can of their available time and money. Often people think what they eat is healthy enough for them, as it has kept them and most people they know going. Many patients assume healthier foods are too expensive and don't want to discuss their financial state. And some patients with health problems that most doctors would assume are primarily related to diet actually eat more "healthily" than I do when I check their food diaries.

Questions doctors could ask that would elicit more helpful information would be along the lines of, "Do you eat breakfast? What do you normally have?" "What are your favorite snacks?" "Do you eat meals sitting down?" and "What is your usual eating routine?" Giving your doctor a two- or three-day food diary can be very helpful, including a short list of favorite foods you don't currently want to give up. Emphasizing the timing and types of food rather than worrying about calories or how much junk food you eat will take off some of the judgment pressure. Calorie counting and basal metabolic rate calculation might be helpful eventually, if simple adjustments don't start moving in the direction of the intended outcome—but not the first time you talk about food. An atmosphere of assumed judgment will only encourage you to be less accurate in your diary.

So, what kinds of food choices are we talking about? The simple "eat from the edges of the grocery store" or "don't eat anything from a bottle, box, can, jar, or bag" sounds like a suggestion for educated, upper middle-class people and might alienate those who aren't. It's better to aim for specific changes that go along with the already existing pattern, maybe changing breakfast first, and changing or eliminating certain snacks. Big and fast changes can derail family routines, leading to arguments from spouses or children, so gentle integration is key.

In my practice, I spend many hours with patients looking for ways to change their diets to be more plant-based, more sustainable, and more enjoyable. Many patients have come to me asking about the latest, greatest diet they'd read so much about, convinced it would cure what ailed them. Many patients seem to be "allergic" to so many foods it is hard to even make suggestions, due partly to their symptoms but also due to their fear of creating more symptoms. A few patients are on diets that have been proven over and over to be harmful long term, but they are quite evangelical that the diet they decided on was the best diet for them and should be adopted by everyone. It was harder to have these discussions before recent studies came out to back up what I'd been saying for years; now the evidence is finally coming around to common sense and pushing us away from alarmist marketing messages.

Not surprisingly, my training in nutrition has been almost entirely outside of medical school. Contrary to popular belief, doctors *do* get a little bit of nutritional training, and it is likely even better nowadays. But it's still incomplete and impractical, heavy on biochemistry and vitamins, and is directed towards things like the DASH[137] diet, which focuses heavily on salt intake, and basic diabetes education around carbohydrates and blood sugar. The majority of my food knowledge I have found out on my own, reading research papers and books by authors with all kinds of backgrounds. I have also taken formal classes and have spoken to dieticians and nutritionists I've met along the way. Learning how to cook was a revelation in itself. And, a large chunk of what I learned about food and cooking was a direct result of getting to know farmers personally.

Probably 50 percent of my reason for investigation was selfish: I felt ill much of the time since I was around eight years old, and my family seems to have terrible genetic predispositions. I wanted to be healthier and prevent real illness for myself down the line. I experimented for years and years; I was vegetarian for almost two decades, had a stretch where I was "gluten-free," and briefly experimented with a diet high in tiny oily fish.[138] For six months or so I ate lots of raw food, then, when that went badly, I spent a few years eating cooked and heavily-spiced food during my full-on Ayurveda phase. I've gone "flour-free" to decrease processed foods and tried a few months of eating 90 percent local. I even went through a nearly "paleo" phase to see if fewer vegetables would feel better to my digestion. Over time, and with the input of good science, I have come to a few conclusions that might be helpful.

Food Basics

First, the human omnivorous digestive system is quite amazing. I'm so impressed that I threw all those different diets at my GI system and I could still function and have enough energy for living! Our digestive systems are able to quickly produce different enzymes, and our gut flora can change in as little as thirty hours to accommodate a change in diet, to ensure we still get adequate nutrition from whatever is available. Surprising to me was that some of the regimens made me feel unexpectedly terrible—especially the gluten-free weeks and the tiny fish, strangely enough. The idea that certain popular diets are "good" for anyone in particular is entirely subjective—and some are clearly *not* good. Food choices need to be individualized, but there are still some reliable underlying guidelines to help people make choices that can improve their nutrition and health.

After combing the most recent research and reading through arguments for and against many different dietary options, there are some themes that remain consistent:

- The amount of variables attached to digestion and energy use is huge, so diets need to be highly individualized. New research on the microbiome will become increasingly helpful in developing effective ones.[139] [140]
- Plants are universally helpful in preventing and reversing illness.
- Whole grain and legume intake is consistently associated with reduction in chronic diseases like diabetes and high cholesterol, and with decreased risk of intestinal cancers.
- Superfoods are generally a marketing myth, and fads can contribute to environmental destruction and economic problems in the parts of the world where they are "discovered."
- Food choices that are environmentally sustainable are dependably healthier.
- Not every "healthy food" is healthy for everyone.
- Community and local, mostly-plant eating is best.[141]
- Fad diets for sure don't work.[142] (To learn more about the health effects of specific diet fads, see appendix 2.)

1. The Holy Grail of Whole Grains

We've become accustomed to refined grains because they make bread softer, sweeter, and easier to texturize and process while keeping shelf life much longer. Why it's a bad idea is easy to grasp, and our cultural appreciation for more diverse tastes and textures needs to be re-expanded. A whole grain is a seed. It has a fibrous outer coating with protein and trace minerals called the *bran* to protect it from predators' digestion and from being destroyed before it has a chance to sprout. The *germ* contains vitamins, minerals, phytochemicals, proteins, and fats. The *endosperm* contains starch, simple proteins, and small amounts of vitamins and soluble fiber for the baby plant to have energy to grow underground and push up to find the sunlight to make its own food.

In our current agricultural system, a huge amount of grain is grown at once and distributed over long distances. This means we need to store it for a long time. But time works against fresh fats and nutrients, since fats tend to oxidize and taste "off," and nutrients degrade and lose value the longer the harvested part of a plant sits around. Refining the grain takes the carbohydrate away from the vitamins and fats that oxidize and taste "off" when left on a shelf for long. And, if the grain is also bleached, its shelf life becomes exponentially longer. This is the case for wheat, corn, rice, and many other grains that can be made into flour.

A Bit of Grain History

In the middle ages, refined flour seemed to be healthier than unrefined, since the earliest versions of the refining process prevented fungi from harming grains stored for long periods of time, preventing some deadly mold-related illnesses. Refined white wheat flour also creates especially delicious tastes and textures like baguettes and cakes, so for cooking and keeping food tasty longer, refining grain was a boon for the food industry. Since refining also makes the sugars easier to digest, the quicker taste of sugar on our tongues also naturally makes us want more.

Over time, refining became more and more efficient; at the same time, grains were being bred to be increasingly heavy in starch.

When vitamins started to be seriously studied in the early 20th century, there was concern around the milling process for flour that removed most of the vitamin content of the grain. During the Great Depression, the economic difficulties pulled nutritional deficiencies into stark relief, and a push to enrich grains ended up in a federal mandate to enrich all white flour.[143] The industry was concerned that since the old milling techniques led to less tasty and worse textured flours, if they went back to making whole grain flour or added back in the actual fiber and germ, they would suffer economically from products with a shorter shelf life and less cake-like textures. So, in order to keep a "healthy" label on their products, the added vitamins were kept as a voluntary process even after the mandate was lifted.

The problem with this system seems obvious, nutritionally. If you eat only the simplest carbohydrates and proteins out of the grain, you lose most of the vitamins, healthy plant fats, the highest quality protein, and the fiber. Adding back in artificial vitamins and alternate types of fiber piecemeal may prevent the worst of nutrition-related diseases, but does not give us a nutritionally equivalent product. This is especially true since many vitamins and the combined action of plant chemicals and vitamins have yet to be understood. In particular, many vitamins require fats to be absorbed into the body, so adding back certain vitamins may not even help, as in the case of GMO "golden rice" and vitamin A.[144]

The things that make grains difficult to keep for months on a shelf are the very things we need to keep our arteries clear, our brains working well, and our bodies strong. Study after study confirms that people who eat whole grains have much less obesity, diabetes, and cancers, which means a logical argument against eating whole grains doesn't exist.[145 146 147 148 149 150 151 152] Eating whole grains helps lower blood pressure, regulates insulin metabolism, protects against cancer, and helps feed and regulate our gut bacteria. Refined grains have none of these benefits, cause the carbohydrate to be absorbed quickly and be stored as fat, and contribute to an extensive list of health problems.

Now, to those with celiac disease, I promise I'm not forgetting you, but rather I encourage you to eat whole grains other than those containing gluten. Eating gluten-free processed foods made of other types of refined flour may keep your symptoms at bay nicely, but will not do your overall health any favors long term. For those of you with symptoms of food sensitivities but *not* celiac disease, the same applies but doesn't relate directly to gluten. Giving up processed foods in general seems to ease symptoms in a large number of people with food sensitivities. Instead of giving up gluten, the added health benefits of eating more whole grains instead of refined grain flours may help your immune system and microbiome work in better harmony.

A secondary but important point here also applies to the subsequent subchapter on fruits and vegetables: try eating more "older" and "wilder" grains. Non-mainstream subspecies of grains don't necessarily have higher nutritional value (although many do, such as red corn versus white corn), but many have different nutrient and taste profiles and may be more enjoyable. This may mean they are trickier to find, but some species are higher in vitamins and phytonutrients and are well worth experimenting with.

An argument I hear quite a bit against grains is that the gradual breeding of the major grains like rice, corn, and wheat have made them too carbohydrate heavy to be healthy for humans in any form. I disagree, since most of the studies have been done on our modern grains, and the results still come out as beneficial for health because of their high fiber and nutrient content. Humans have been eating grains for millennia, while food sensitivities are very new and largely confined to those in the rich, Western nations. This suggests other factors are more heavily implicated than the whole grains themselves. If you favor trying more grains with a higher ratio of nutrients to carbohydrates, such as green corn, rye, or buckwheat, go for it, since it certainly makes the flavors more interesting and cooking more exciting![153]

In any case, the point about "whole" applies to all grains. Refining legumes and "ancient" grains into flour still breaks down cell walls and allows the sugars to be digested much faster. Processing at high temperatures, which is universally the case for processed foods, changes structure of carbohydrates, fats, and nutrients and causes bitterness and strange textures to occur. We're not sure yet how our body responds to these changes in food molecule structure, and as far as I know, no longitudinal studies have been performed in this area. Also, just like your average white flour, refining grains and beans often simply rids them of many of their nutritious components that are distinct from those found in fruits and vegetables and the key to the health benefits of these foods.

Read labels on the processed food you decide to buy, and beware of "health claims" and fads. When it says "whole grain" or "ancient grains" on the package, there might be just a tiny percentage of whole grains in the food. If enriched white flour is one of the first ingredients in a long list, this means refined white flour with artificial vitamins added back in is really what you're purchasing. The added bits don't increase the nutritional value enough to justify the additional price they can charge for the health claim.

Along the same lines, countries far from the U.S. that have traditionally grown a food which has now become a popular fad may have their economies and communities disrupted by a sudden spike in demand from developed nations with huge consumer power. A good example is quinoa in Bolivia, where the increased demand for its export has raised the prices for the local poor population and encouraged non-native farming methods that degrade the soil, causing conflict within the traditional community structure.[154] While it may settle out all right in the end and benefit the traditional farmers eventually, the economic shock was not justified by the fad's health claims.

While quinoa is higher in protein than most grains and is a very hearty plant that can be grown in arid environments, the change in demand has definitely not all been positive. There are fair trade options available, as far as that goes, but it can also be grown in the U.S. It is good to remember that a colorful corn added to beans is also a high protein option and, with other vegetables added, makes a much more colorful, nutrient-dense, and exciting plate of food than only quinoa. As always, it is important to be educated about where your food comes from, and when possible, try to make ethical decisions about the kind of food system your money will be supporting.

Another note about the farmers—many foods high in nutritional value can be grown right in our backyards, depending on where we live in the country. The U.S. climate is diverse enough that pretty much anything we decide we want to eat can be grown in at least one of our states. Depending on each person's economic status, making decisions that are more helpful to farmers, the soil, air, and water is possible to varying extents. Whole grains that have been grown without pesticides and fungicides, as fresh and as close to you as possible to preserve their nutrient content, and that are highest in nutritional value are better for you, the farmers, and the environment.

2. Plants Really Are the Answer

First, Vegetables

If you grew up in the U.S., your parents probably tried constantly to get you to eat more vegetables. Most of us can remember fighting our parents about one or more varieties we had temporarily declared inedible. Even my grandparents, one of whom grew up in a depression-era home of six children without his father and the other in an orphanage, seemed to be prepared for each argument, as if they grew up experiencing the same sort of conflicts themselves. Some of this may be due to the bitter taste present in many vegetables, which children rarely appreciate, and some people actually have a genetic predisposition to detest bitterness. Bitter taste receptors have been found not just on our tongues, but also in our GI tracts, lungs, sinuses, and even inside the testes! To me, this means the use of bitter herbs and substances as medicines for millennia is not surprising, nor is the unpleasantness of the flavor in large quantities. The old adage that anything is a medicine or a poison depending on dose seems very clear in the case of substances that have a bitter taste.

But bitter is just one of the taste clues to many a vegetable's health benefits, and it turns out that some of the most bitter vegetables are the best at staving off diabetes and are highest in antioxidants and phytochemicals that prevent cancer. Over the past few hundred years, and the last 30 in particular, bitterness and other tastes like sourness and astringency have been gradually bred out of many of our standard fruits and vegetables, eliminating not just some of the more complex flavors in favor of simple sweetness, but also some of the healthiest nutrients. Despite selective breeding to increase sugar content and decrease nutritional value, eating more fruits and vegetables along with nuts and seeds is still consistently and firmly associated with improved health, particularly in people with chronic diseases like diabetes and heart disease.[155] [156] [157]

While starchy tubers and grains make up the most calories of the majority of indigenous diets, and many incorporate meat, plant foods have always been humans' mainstay of phytonutrients, fiber, and taste variety. Our flatter teeth favor grinding rather than ripping to swallow whole (the way pure carnivores' only sharp teeth do), and our digestive tracts are comparatively long. This indicates mostly herbivore behavior in our history. More recently, our large intestines (where most herbivores have to ferment—i.e., cook!—large amounts of plant matter with the help of specialized bacteria) have shortened, while our small intestines lengthened, likely because we started cooking, which made it easier to get nutrients from our food.[158] [159]

Feeding our gut bacteria is a necessary priority, and eating more vegetables and fruits helps by contributing more fiber and phytochemicals.[160] We also know there are a variety of studies that prove diets with high percentages of plant foods are better for most of us, promoting longevity and preventing cancer, diabetes, heart disease, and obesity.[161] [162] [163] [164] From journalist Jo Robinson and her book *Eating on the Wild Side*, we also know that some vegetables and fruits are healthiest cooked, and some healthiest raw or lightly cooked.[165] Whether cooking or eating raw vegetables, remember to add a small amount of healthy fat to help absorb fat-requiring vitamins like A, D, E, and K.

Trying to get around eating actual vegetables by taking pills or other shortcuts doesn't produce the effects of actually eating the food. Juicing, while hugely popular, does not meet this criteria at all, especially when processed sugar like cane and agave are used to sweeten a more sour or vegetable-heavy mix. Similarly, vegetable protein isolates, like the type that are used in energy bars and supplements, can actually have negative effects on health. Multiple studies a few years ago warned about the negative effects of soy protein supplements, but eating whole food soy such as tofu, tempeh, miso, and soymilk in normal amounts seems to always be beneficial.[166]

It is absolutely true that not all of us have the luxury to make food choices that can be more expensive, difficult to find, or require more time to cook. However, there are still general principles that can help anyone improve their nutrition intake with more vegetables, no matter what the circumstances are. SNAP benefits are now accepted at many farmers' markets, food banks often can accept unsold food from farmers' markets, physicians are writing prescriptions for CSA boxes, and even some hospitals are adding fresh food from local farms or their own gardens to "hospital food;" the cultural shift towards making sure fresh healthy food is available to everyone is clearly catching on.

For people who like *this* kind of book, I'd like to also recommend checking out two other books: *The Jungle Effect* by Daphne Miller, MD, and *Eating on the Wild Side*, by Jo Robinson.[167] [168] *The Jungle Effect* is a great resource to start with, especially if you have a genetic predisposition to one of the most common chronic diseases or cancers. Miller is a great writer and illustrates nicely how different ancient and traditional diet principles can be modified to modern versions to help reverse problems like depression and diabetes. Robinson's book is wonderful, too. She takes plant groups and gives examples of how to prepare them to best nutritional effect and also explains which varieties have the highest nutritional content. This will help you seek out new vegetables to try and make sure you prepare them to best effect.

Fruit with Fiber versus Fruit Sugar

For tens of thousands of years, fruits were eaten seasonally, in binges, when each variety was available. I imagine fruits used to be the most exciting part of any diet given the high sugar content, brief availability, and likelihood of accidental fermentation! As recently as the early 1900s, an orange in a Christmas stocking was still rare, expensive, and the best present possible. That image stuck with me as something strange and tragic when I saw it as a small child, growing up as I did with oranges and bananas available and expected year round.

Each fruit is naturally only in season for a short time, and overeating whole fruits in a short time period is not usually harmful, except for maybe a bit of rapid digestion. Historically, the tendency to be attracted to sugar hasn't been a problem until now. The breeding of fruits to have higher sugar content for increased sweet taste has led to decreases in nutrition content, and year-round availability due to quick shipping and refrigeration has changed how we consume fruit. This same process has facilitated other starchy foods like potatoes and grains being bred to be larger and sweeter over time, and they are consumed more often, in more processed forms, and in larger quantities now, just like fruit. Flours, juices, fruit concentrates added to foods, and extended shelf life keeps us binging year round, like deer with a windfall of apples in the autumn. Technology has made simple carbohydrates and sugars easier to access than would ever happen in nature, enabling humans' hardwiring for sugar addiction to turn into a worldwide obesity epidemic.

Fruit is high in sugar, which is why it is so delicious. The fiber and nutrients make it a definitely healthy addition to a diet with vegetables and whole grains as its base. However, like "healthy fats," whole fruits still need to be eaten in moderation with attention to fruit type. Fruits like watermelon, with its high water content, and pomegranates, with their

Making Veggies Exciting

If you're like me, and grew up eating primarily processed food, fresh vegetables can be exciting enough without needing any help, except perhaps a sprinkle of salt and pepper and a drizzle of olive oil. But for some people, vegetables are unappealing unless smothered in cheese or sugar, and considering increasing the amount of vegetables might sound repulsive—much like adding an additional canned vegetable serving to my dinner seemed like torture to me growing up in Illinois.

For some people, gardening is the answer, since the joy of preparing and eating something you've grown is nearly universal. But sometimes it's more about preparation and kitchen tricks. There are several books on "hiding" veggies to increase children's intake, but since their suggestions are delicious, they work for adults as well! I also suggest experimenting with raw, cooked, and pickled vegetables, and using new spice mixtures like za'atar or herbes de provence. Although tempting, wrapping them in bacon or cheese or drowning a stir-fry or pasta in sugary sauces works against you. Cooking this way negates many of the benefits of the vegetables, making the meal at best nutritionally neutral.[169]

Also, for children in particular, tastes change frequently. Keep trying things you may not have liked as a child, or even just a few years back, especially if it is prepared differently than you've had before. Just adding something like nutmeg, white pepper, cumin, or a bay leaf can wildly improve the flavor of a sauce, soup, or whole vegetable without even being able to taste the specific flavor of the spice.

irritatingly difficult natural packaging, are difficult to eat in excess when eaten whole. But many other fruits, especially dried fruit or nutritionally weaker varieties, such as yellow peaches, white raspberries, or golden delicious apples, are easier to go overboard with due to their high sugar content.

Too much sugar is still too much sugar, so treat juices and smoothies like you would butter or chocolate. The exception would be, perhaps, as a way to get vitamins into your system if you aren't able to eat solid foods while ill. Again, make sure to go slowly with dried fruit since the sugar:water ratio is high. Finally, to lower your carbon footprint, unless you live in the Caribbean or Hawaii, go easy on fruit from far away like bananas and coconuts.

Overall, the most important point is to eat vegetables and fruits that are whole, with minimal processing. This ensures the highest water content for best digestion and ensures that most of the vitamins and fiber are intact and available for our gut flora to use.

To Meat or Not to Meat?

The various arguments about whether or not to eat meat (and animal products generally) can be boiled down to two main issues: the horrible environmental impact and terrible conditions for animals in modern, large agribusiness (more in chapter 7) and antibiotic resistance. The simplest solution to both of these issues (since most people want to eat at least some meat) is to eat *less* meat, and to choose pastured meat, dairy, and eggs from sources you have researched. There is growing evidence that sustainably farmed animals (in much fewer numbers than we currently consume) can contribute to soil improvement and grassland restoration, and when managed correctly, can perhaps repair environments that have undergone desertification.[170] [171] [172]

As for direct human health effects and food purchasing choices, there are a few helpful things to keep in mind. Eating processed meats and cooking meat at high temperatures are associated with more intestinal cancers, so eating healthy, fresh animal protein and cooking at lower temperatures is important.[173] [174] Antibiotic resistance is a major health concern as well. Around 80 percent by weight of antibiotics sold in the U.S. are used on agriculturally raised animals, including fish, to either increase their weight quickly or to treat infections from living in damaging conditions. This is likely a main cause of most emerging antibiotic resistant infections in humans, especially in light of 2015's news about colistin resistance, which is increasingly worrisome.[175] If animals are allowed to live comfortably and in a more natural social environment with fewer individuals forced close together, antibiotics are needed considerably less frequently.

I should mention dairy specifically here, given that it makes up such a huge part of the "American diet." Dairy is a great source of healthy fat and protein, and even those with lactose intolerance can gradually increase the number of gut bacteria that can digest it. The newest studies suggest that eating a bit of full-fat dairy milk and yogurt is healthy, and that cheese and small amounts of butter don't seem to cause undue harm.[176] Given that dairy production has many of the same issues as meat production (antibiotics, ethical treatment of animals, and the tendency of Americans to overeat fat and protein), it seems that moderation—eat/drink less and eat/drink more plant-based foods—is again the best path to take with dairy.

If we collectively agree to stop breeding animals in order to make them genetically unable to mate or support themselves, with thin bones and heavy breasts in the case of turkeys and chickens, they will also be healthier and less in need of antibiotics and intensive veterinary care. If we collectively favor purchases from small farms, where sick animals are easier to isolate and products are easier to track, food-borne illness outbreaks and animal-to-human outbreaks of viruses like avian and porcine flus will decline and be easier to contain.

3. Cook Your Own Food

Cooking is so key to our health and our survival as a species, it is strange that it has become seemingly optional. Cooking tubers, grains, and vegetables allowed humans easier access to carbohydrates and vitamins than is possible from raw food, so it is cooking that allowed our brains to evolve faster than previously possible.[177] Food expert and journalist Michael Pollan's basic conclusion, after decades of research about food, is that the best thing you can do for your health is to cook your own food.[178] No matter what you choose to eat, if you prepare it yourself, there will be fewer additives, it will be fresher, and at the very least you have a better chance of finding out where it came from and how the ingredients affected the environment as it was grown.

If you've decided for yourself, or if your doctor has told you or someone in your family to "eat better" or "eat more vegetables," figuring out how to do that within current habit patterns might seem difficult. But learning how to cook new foods and more whole foods is something that everyone can benefit from, and is well worth trying. For most of my patients, and for me, improving our diets is best done in baby steps. Jumping feet first into an entirely new set of unfamiliar foods is unnecessarily stressful, especially in a family with many different opinions about food. Changing habit patterns in any area of life works best if one follows evidence-based weight loss recommendations: slow and steady is sustainable and allows reaching long-term goals, while sudden changes are likely to be thrown aside quickly, leading to potentially worse results than one started with. But just one new recipe successfully and deliciously accomplished means more are possible and even likely. Finding one new vegetable that works when added to an old recipe means it might work in another.

Where to Start

We all know that something that comes directly from the earth is better for us than something from a box or package. We know that French fries and candy are on the "bad for us" end of the spectrum. Despite knowing this, we still regularly ignore these seemingly inherent truths and go with our basic impulses to continue to eat food with low nutritional value. And food companies use these predilections to infuse more sugars, salt, and fats to entice us to keep eating this way. Thankfully, our food culture is changing, with more farmers' markets every year, more farm-to-table restaurants, and even large fast food chains like Panera and Wal-Mart beginning to pay attention to the treatment of the animals and land used to produce their food. But when possible, we still need to make the choices—with our votes and our dollars—that help change what

Looking back on my own often-sketchy "food life" growing up in the Midwest, I feel so lucky to have had a mother who cared tremendously about my nutrition, and that I never had to go hungry. I was lucky enough to go away to college and meet people who ate very differently than I had growing up. I have also been privileged to have the chance to decide to be vegetarian for nearly two decades of my life, and then later to decide to again embrace a more omnivorous diet. But my health has not always made it easy to figure out what foods worked for me, and I grew up eating mostly highly processed and pre-packaged foods. I need to emphasize that wherever you are with your health or economic situation, there are ways to improve nutrition without expensive supplements.

is available for the better and keep us healthy in the meantime. Let's dig in.

Here is a list of ways to start making small manageable changes, since even tiny improvements can make a big difference over time.

Cook for yourself more often.

- Eat sitting down.
- Favor ingredients that are bought separately, buy staples in bulk, and reuse containers. You'll learn to estimate how much salt, spices, and other basics you're using, and you can then buy only as much as you need to keep ingredients fresh and avoid waste.
- Use colorful, whole vegetables when creating stir-fries and pasta sauces, and substitute ingredients to experiment.
- Learn to make great soups, so vegetables that might otherwise be on their last legs or thrown out have a new, delicious chance to shine.
- Learn what spices you like best and how to use them to change the flavors of dishes for more variety. Things like turmeric and fresh herbs add nutritional and medicinal value to meals as well as flavor.

Eat more plants, less meat.

- Replace some meat with small sustainable fish (if canned, pick water-packed varieties).
- Cook meat, fish, and fat-containing foods at low temperatures most of the time to reduce cancer risk.
- Sustainable fish and pasture-raised and -finished meat are healthy additions in small amounts for most people.[179]

Eat as little processed food as you can manage.

- Eat more whole grains, with all their nutrients and fiber.
- Eat more whole plants, including legumes—not fried or with added sugar.
- Particularly avoid sugar in liquid form (store-bought drinks, processed sauces, and dressings) and in flour products (cookies, packaged breads, and cakes). In these products, sugar is harder to notice and is often paired with excess salt and fat; it's also ingested and digested far more quickly than in whole food form.

Learn what you can easily grow and grow some of your own food.

- Gardening is great for your microbiome and can save you money by growing expensive or easily perishable veggies like tomatoes and leafy greens, even in pots inside near a window or outside near your door. If you get really into it, check in with urban farming classes and master gardeners in your town.
- Fresh herbs can be grown in your kitchen, making it easy and economical to add nutritional value and freshness to soups, salads, and stir-fries.
- Help native bees! Grow flowering plants and food, especially ones native to your area, and never use sprays or buy seeds or plants pre-sprayed.
- Start composting if you have room or if your city has a program. And if you do have a lawn, don't spray it! Leave those dandelions and clover—bees love them. Or consider an even more bug and bee-friendly ground cover.

Buy local.

- Buy from local farmers when possible, and find and support those who use sustainable practices. (Of course, not all local farming is sustainable, so use good judgment and pick your battles wisely.[180] [181] [182] [183]) Even if you only buy less expensive, sustainably-grown staples like onions and potatoes from your nearest farmers' market, you will help local farmers stay solvent and support clean local soil and water.

- When buying products from a grocery store, check the labels; it might be easier to find out how workers and the land are treated in your state than in Asia or South America.

- Buy organic/sustainable when possible. Prioritize buying organic vegetables and fruits that have a high requirement for and ability to absorb pesticides and fungicides, such as strawberries, stone fruit, and tomatoes.[184] [185] Give yourself a break if you need to buy conventionally grown foods that don't require as many sprays or fertilizers, like avocados, brassica vegetables, and garlic.[186]

Eat with your community.

Blue Zones, local food, and sustainability is what chapter 7 is all about.

Social connections in general are getting more attention in research related to food and longevity. "Blue Zones" are associated with particular dietary patterns, but most of these case studies involve community rituals around eating together and health activities enjoyed in the local culture.[187] Even *Time* magazine recently ran a popular article on social connections, citing research on longevity and illness differences between those with few versus many close friends and family.[188]

Taking advantage of the benefits of community is as simple as eating regularly with family or friends and involving others in the process of meal preparation. If you often eat alone, make sure to enjoy what you eat and cook for yourself as you would for a dear friend. Keep in contact with family and friends and enjoy time with people with similar interests, while making room for diversity and learning from people with different views and cultural preferences.

6

OUR BUGS ARE OUR REASON FOR LIVING

New research on our gut microbiome is really exciting right now for the medical community and also for those with intestinal and immune problems. Medical professionals are finally coming to understand that the ecosystem in and around our surfaces (intestines, skin, vaginas, teeth, etc.) doesn't just house a huge number of passive passengers—the microbes we carry with us train our immune systems, make neurotransmitters and hormones, digest our food, help us fight infection, and influence how we process each calorie we eat and whether we will gain weight or remain at a healthy weight.[189] [190] [191] [192] [193] [194] The interactions between our bacteria, food, and nervous and immune systems are delicate and amazing. There are even studies looking at tailoring probiotics, antibiotics, and food lists to the genetics of our microbiomes.[195] [196]

This is a huge philosophical paradigm shift and a cornerstone of the concept of Sustainable Health. We are traveling at light speed away from the standpoint we've had since the discovery of bacteria—that "bugs are the enemy"—and realizing how intricately we are connected to and dependent on the bugs that live in, on, and around us. This is exactly the type of thinking that illustrates our interrelatedness with the environment that the entire medical field would do well to embrace.

How Our Allies Work With Us: Bugs For Your Birthday

The day we are born, microbial allies start colonizing us. It's best if we get to travel down our mother's birth canal in a normal exit position (face down, towards her rectum, in case you were wondering). Our entrance is greeted by microbes that stick to our skin, our mucous membranes, and are swallowed right away to start multiplying in our intestines.[197] [198] [199] These new tenants in our guts start training our immune systems immediately. The lactobacilli in our mother's vaginal canal increase dramatically right before birth, and the increased numbers we take in on our way out help us digest our very first meal, which, containing milk sugars, feeds them at the same time. Mother's milk contains perfect nutrition, including more bacteria to help us digest, and oligosaccharides *we* can't digest that are solely there to feed our newly acquired gastrointestinal friends, whom we need to break down breast milk components for energy and nutrition.[200]

In addition, to assist building our immune systems, our mother's body makes antibodies for us in utero and later sends them through breast milk.[201] [202] If a baby catches a cold, beyond just being exposed like anyone else nearby through baby slobber and proximity, the vacuum created when the baby breastfeeds seems to allow a wee bit of backwash so the mother's immune system gets exposed to the virus as well, and can then make antibodies and deliver them to the baby in the milk.[203] It's a pretty impressive system.

Everything that happens in these first few hours and months of life dramatically affects our immune system for the rest of our lives.[204] Lack of good bacterial exposure early on can predispose us to obesity, asthma, juvenile rheumatoid arthritis, inflammatory bowel disease, immune deficiency, cumulative trauma disorders, and even leukemia.[205] There is also new research on whether antibiotics given to mothers before birth affects microbial diversity in their children and therefore immune function. Doctors recognizing these connections have started to study whether it would improve C-section babies' immune exposure at birth to wipe them down with their mother's vaginal secretions.[206] [207] A "dirtier" birth (meaning your average uncomplicated vaginal birth with decent exposure to mother's bacterial colonies) is good for babies' health for the rest of their lives. This suggests long-term health outcomes could be improved with simple practices like immediate skin-to-skin contact (especially for preterm infants), bedside sleepers for easy access to feeding during the night, and avoidance of neonatal cleansing when possible.

Mud Pies and Animal Friends Are Really Good for You

As we grow up, exposure to animals, dirt, and sick older siblings seems to protect us from allergies, asthma, and skin disorders.[208] [209] [210] [211] This makes sense since the more exposure our immune systems get to different types of bacteria, viruses, and worms, the better it is at distinguishing what is harmful to us and what is helpful. It's also worth noting that children from countries who spend more time outside have significantly different microbial profiles, but it is still unknown exactly what all these bacteria do and what health benefits and downsides each correlate with.[212] It is certain that more diversity is better, though, just as diversity is critical in every natural ecosystem. Even our appendix is more important than we thought, since it is a huge repository of bacteria and lymph tissue, and likely plays an essential role in how our immune system communicates with our microbiome. It may even be responsible for repopulating our gut after an illness wreaks havoc on our bacterial balance.[213] We may find that if not overwhelmed by infection, the appendix is a lot more helpful than we thought.

When we get an infection in the course of everyday life, our immune systems bounce back, repair damaged intestinal, bronchial, and sinus mucosal linings, and our healthy microbial and immune systems rebuild themselves, now with new knowledge of a "bad" type of invader. As miraculous and life saving as antibiotics can be, they are only vaguely selective about what they kill, and routinely take out around one third of our "good" bacteria along with the "bad" that caused the illness in the first place.[214] This mass annihilation of our microbial friends lasts around three months, sometimes longer, affecting digestion and immunity.[215 216 217 218]

Antibiotics can make it more likely for us to get the flu, and can make us more susceptible to things like rotavirus by harming the good bacteria that help our immune systems fight off pathogens.[219 220] Since our microbiome is so intimately connected to our immune systems, it isn't surprising that autoimmune diseases like Crohn's disease are definitely linked to, if not caused by, antibiotic exposure.[221] Antibiotics have other side effects too, some we are just beginning to understand, including nerve and tendon damage, hallucinations, and cardiovascular events.[222] This is troubling, since antibiotics intended for serious infections are still routinely given for things like viral colds, coughs, and ear infections, even though this is against current recommendations.[223]

Even more worrying is that the vast majority of the antibiotics used in the U.S. are given to livestock, often daily, for prevention of illnesses that run rampant through overcrowded and unnatural farm conditions, as well as to increase weight gain.[224 225] The resulting resistant infections from consistent overuse of antibiotics end up affecting humans as well as wild animals.[226 227 228] These links are finally being noticed in the mainstream media as evidenced by the coverage of the colistin resistance cases that started appearing in the early 2010s. Less dramatic, but no less of an issue, there is now evidence that antibiotics may directly cause weight gain in humans, due to disruption of healthy flora and selection for bacteria that might be extra good at wringing extra calories from food.[229]

Beyond antibiotics, our obsession with cleanliness means that we use products in our homes and on our bodies that kill many bacteria, but may also be causing our internal microbiomes harm. Chemicals to extend shelf life in fast food and processed food, as well as to kill bacteria on our skin or on household surfaces, may be doing much more harm than good, especially in the case of additives like triclosan.[230] [231] [232] Parabens have also been the subject of several studies, since they are antimicrobial and can act as endocrine disruptors and have been found not just in products to extend shelf life, but in food and in the bodies of 95 percent of people.[233] [234] Since some of these chemicals don't break down for 50 years or more, and they are found in wastewater, their toxic effect on wildlife will likely last ages, even if we manage to ban all the ones we've identified as harmful.[235] Even the International Federation of Gynecologists and Obstetrics have made statements about banning endocrine disruptors, including those found in plastics.[236]

Extending out of our homes to our farms, which I'll talk more about in the next chapter, glycophosphate, one of the most common pesticides used in agriculture, has been absorbed by humans and causes helpful bacteria to die (lactobacillus and bifidobacteria), but pathogenic bacteria (clostridium and salmonella) are resistant.[237] Since humans living near farms are exposed often, as of course are farmworkers applying the pesticide, long-term mild exposure may be causing problems that the available studies conducted by the chemical companies have so far missed.

Genetic manipulation may also prove to be harmful in some cases in ways we can't predict. Genes added to plants to produce a toxic chemical to kill insects have been found in animals who eat the plants—and in humans—and we have no idea what the side effects might be over time.[238] It may seem like a small thing for a bit of bug-killing toxin to be found in people's blood. It might not be worrying that a bit of a chemical that keeps our shampoo fresh for several years could act like a hormone. But most of us absorb a little of *many* of these products every day, from lotions, soaps, other household products, and from our food. The cumulative effect of things individually generally recognized as "safe" by the FDA may eventually be found to be truly harmful to our microbiome, to our complicated hormonal system, and to the environment around us.

We already know that puberty, menopause, and pregnancy alter our microbiome,[239] that gut bacteria influence estrogen,[240] and that food and supplement products that include estrogen-like compounds in high concentrations affect fertility and reproductive cancers.[241] [242] It stands to reason that absorbing even small amounts of hormone-like substances over time may change the feedback mechanism with our gut bacteria and our endocrine system. It would not surprise me at all if we soon find that exposure to some of these chemical disruptors of our

In one of the most astonishing (to me) studies I read, researchers took bacteria from male mice's intestines and transferred them to immature female mice at genetic risk for type 1 diabetes.[243] The female mice had consistently high testosterone levels long after the transplant and were protected from type 1 diabetes, suggesting that not only did the transfer bacteria take up residence happily without their immature systems kicking them out, but the new microflora also protected the little mice by working with their hormonal and immune systems to prevent autoimmunity, despite their genetic susceptibility and opposite genetic gender. This particular study doesn't explain the mechanisms of how it worked, but it does firm up the association between a healthy microbiome and hormonal balance and function, as well as the relatively new idea that the immune system in our guts works with our endocrine system and can predispose us to or prevent serious immune dysfunction.

microbiomes are common contributing causes of early puberty, infertility, and reproductive cancers.

There are a myriad of interesting studies on human illnesses and gut flora, and although many show solid correlations, none have yet cut through the complexity of our immune/microbiome/diet/neurologic/hormonal system to give good answers on how to definitively prevent or treat any of these issues. We also know that our gut flora are important in epigenetics, modulating which genes turn on and off. It makes sense that if we have less than healthy lifestyles and diets, which encourage less beneficial microbial friends and decreased microbial diversity, then we may be increasing the chances that the "disease-producing" genes will get turned on rather than stay off. This can lead to development of diseases we were genetically predisposed to, but which we may otherwise not have developed.

Despite the complexity we're uncovering, some interesting new info can point us in possible positive therapeutic directions:

- Certain bacteria are found at lower concentrations in inflammatory bowel disease (IBD) patients. A possible reason is a disruption in mineral absorption and production of growth factor in the intestines.[244] This could mean that a targeted probiotic supplement might be of help.
- A severe bout of a viral stomach flu may help set off IBD,[245] [246] along with a host of other risk factors from patients' environment, lifestyle, and related illness-causing bugs.[247]
- Drugs like ibuprofen, genetic predisposition, foods, infections, psychological stress, and other risk factors for irritable bowel syndrome (IBS) have been reported, leading to successful use of elimination diets and stress-reduction-based symptom improvements in some patients.[248] [249]

Eventually these puzzle pieces could help with treatment of symptoms or help us prevent symptoms by identifying genetically susceptible patients. For instance, L-carnitine from meat is turned into artery-clogging TMAO (trimethylamine-N-oxide) by gut bacteria.[250] It may be helpful for patients who carry more of the offending type of gut bacteria to avoid meat. A recent study suggested that obesity might be actually "caught" from or perpetuated by close friends, possibly by exchange of flora due to simple frequent proximity.[251] This means that the reverse may be true as well, allowing us to treat groups of friends and families together more effectively.

Another mechanism operating in overweight people may be that different microflora might be causing us to crave certain foods that improve survival. A study on toxoplasmosis (most people know it as the parasitic protozoa found in cat litter that pregnant women need to avoid) showed mice infected with toxoplasma were attracted to cat urine (bad for the mice, great for toxoplasmosis' life cycle). This study has been covered in a number of articles, including my favorite one on Radiolab.[252] [253] Though obviously we aren't mice and clearly aren't attracted to cat urine, a similar effect may be happening more subtly with our gut bacteria, which constantly speak to our enteric nervous system (ENS), or our "second brain" as it is often referred to. We've only recently discovered that our bacteria make neurotransmitters that affect our nervous and immune systems.[254] [255] [256] [257] Two of our main neurotransmitters, serotonin and dopamine, affect feelings of well-being and contentment, among many other functions. Most of our serotonin is produced in our intestines, along with huge amounts of dopamine and other neurotransmitters. Since more messages go up from our intestines through the vagus nerve to our brains than come back down, it's likely we've only just scratched the surface of our bacteria's communication expertise.[258] [259]

At this point, it's very clear that our gut bacteria affect our health alongside our mood, even if we're not yet sure exactly how, why, how to help, or in which cases the microbiome is the cause or just one part of the symptom web.[260] But there are a number of studies showing promise for figuring out more of the puzzle:

- It seems higher percentages of certain bacteria (campylobacter, in this case) are associated with depressive behavior in mice (which also may encourage them to eat more).[261]
- When monkeys are stressed by being separated from their mothers, there is a decrease in helpful flora and they are more susceptible to infection.[262] [263]
- In nervous mice, giving them microflora from adventurous mice makes them more adventurous too, and affects neurotransmitter activity in the hippocampus.[264]
- Certain bacteria create intestinal pain when certain nutrients are absent, possibly controlling our food cravings through pain.
- Yet another study found that certain bacteria are necessary for pain sensitivity, which may help explain different people's pain perception levels in many illnesses.[265] [266]

This entire field is wide open for more study, and the potential for finding helpful treatments is vast.

Probiotics: Helpful or Just Band-Aids?

A probiotic is a supplement made of specific strains of microorganisms delivered as a medicinal dose with the intention of affecting the intestinal microbiome. Probiotics have become a hugely profitable industry for supplement companies. Unfortunately, very few probiotics actually contain what is listed on their labels, since the FDA still doesn't regulate supplements. Many contain strains that haven't been proven to help *anyone*, much less been proven to be the panacea the companies claim. It sounds like a great idea to take a few million bacteria in a pill that might colonize you and help your digestion and general health, but we have trillions of bacteria that have already fought to maintain a spot in our gut. These inhabitants have already "discussed" their location and function with our immune and neurologic systems, and replicate furiously all day and all night. Taking a pill of "newbies" who aren't currently included in the mix might just cause a bit of diarrhea rather than ousting any particular pathogens or joining forces with our allies.

Bacteria don't work singly anyway; in concert with other microbes they work with the immune and nervous systems, the digestive system, and with incoming food that feeds both them and us. Just like monocrop agriculture is risky and promotes terrible soil conditions, I can't imagine it is any different in our own "gut gardens," making the case shaky for large repeated doses of any one strain. It's difficult to isolate enough variables to be certain which, if any, one strain would be helpful for any individual.

Many studies on probiotics have shown correlations with certain strains and improved symptoms,[267] [268] [269] [270] [271] [272] [273] [274] but while probiotics seem to help in some cases, most reviews are still inconclusive since the results vary so much.[275] [276] [277] [278] Probiotics don't usually cause harmful side effects, with the notable exception of some people immunocompromised from severe illness, cancer, or surgery, who developed life-threatening infections from probiotics.[279] [280] A newer study is worrying in that it showed that taking probiotics after a gastrointestinal illness might slow down our own healthy bacteria from repopulating our gut lining. [281]

Probiotics prescribed by your doctor are usually the strains that have been tested and proven helpful for specific illnesses like ulcerative colitis or during antibiotic use. They need to be continually administered because none so far seem to last after halting supplementation. Some doctors recommend taking them daily from 90 days to two years to see effects, depending on the reason for the prescription, but to me this means they may not be healing the underlying problem, and at best should be used as an adjunctive treatment with more extensive diet and lifestyle changes.

As we've seen, there are a huge number of variables in the complex system of our gut ecology inside the complex system of our bodies, situated in the complex system of our environment, culture, and history. This means that although some probiotics might be helpful, they are at this point mostly just a "drop in the ocean." To change a system that is out of balance, it's unlikely a "pill" will fix problems that are almost always multi-factorial. This isn't to say probiotics might not be found to be a key part in a treatment plan for a variety of illnesses, but pre-biotic foods, pro-biotic foods, and highly nutritious foods need to be included as well (see chapter 5). When a relatively healthy person changes their diet, gut bacterial profiles can change within a day, no probiotics necessary.[282]

But in some patients that suffer from celiac disease, even after a long-term, gluten-free diet, their uncomfortable symptoms still persist and their intestinal bacterial profiles stubbornly remain weighted toward less helpful microbes.[283] Even stranger, newer research on strains of bacteria that have been previously identified as "definitely bad," like *Helicobacter pylori*, actually may protect us from certain types of inflammation-induced cancers.[284] The complexity is such that even melatonin (as you'll remember from chapter 4) may prove to be a mediator for how well a probiotic works.[285]

It's best to keep in mind that if your system is stressed and your microbial diversity is low or out of balance, taking a probiotic pill or starting to eat different foods suddenly can, rather than helping, cause more uncomfortable symptoms. Try one new thing at a time, for long enough to allow your body to complete a few monthly hormonal cycles, so any daily and monthly changes in microbes will get acclimated to the new additions.

If you decide to try probiotics or are prescribed them, make sure the brand legitimately contains what it claims to. Then start slowly and take them for a good length of time—at least three to six months—before deciding whether they have helped. If you want to stop taking them, taper off, so as not to upset the new balance they have achieved.

Someone Else's Poo!

What is heartening is that some of the most serious problems linked with disruptions in healthy flora can be reversed, sometimes by administering "someone else's poo" (yes, I'm talking about fecal transplants), or even giving patients "pathogenic" organisms. Fecal transplants are now considered a definitive treatment for the resistant form of antibiotic-related diarrhea called *C. difficile* (often called C-diff). There might be other applications of this idea as more studies are done on humans. For instance, obese mice given thin mice's gut flora lose weight, and vice versa.[286] [287] Even stranger, giving worms to Crohn's patients may reset the immune system and reverse the disease,[288] [289] and a strain of brewers' yeast may be better than one common antibiotic for Giardia treatment.[290] [291] Science is still rather at the blunt stage of "let's try this seemingly random thing," since our knowledge is incomplete, but we seem to be edging closer to very promising, if odd-sounding, effective gut flora treatments!

In the Gut of the Beholder

All of this means we don't have nearly enough information to make sweeping statements about what is "good" and what is "bad" for us as far as gut bacteria species, treatments for illnesses, and even *causes* of illnesses. It's interesting to me that in the current craze created by the new research proving how important our personal microbiome is, physicians (and marketing professionals) have latched onto it as "finding the root cause" of illnesses. The problem with this thinking is that with a complex system, there may not be only one "root cause." The best health regimens are "in the gut of the beholder," not in what the latest fad proponent believes.

Making things more complicated, a person's microbiome is at least partly passed down through generations, with each consecutive generation having less diversity, especially if low fiber and low nutrition diets persist. Changing the diet of a third generation descendent with the least gut diversity in the family doesn't seem to allow the system to recover: but fecal transplants do.[292] To me this makes more sense as to why diet changes only help about a third of people, and for others, the changes either make no difference or worsen symptoms. The rule of thirds from Eastern medicine (every treatment will help a third, harm a third, and not effect a third of those treated) seems to apply to even the newest research findings.

In general though, a few things seem to be dependably helpful:

- Microbiome diversity and being "dirtier" is associated with health.[293] [294] [295] [296] [297] [298] Transplanting a healthy person's diverse microbiome can save the lives of people with severe infections or some autoimmune illnesses.
- Plant-based diets are associated with a microbiome profile that is associated with health, even in people genetically predisposed to a severe illness like Prader-Willi syndrome.[299]
- Coping strategies for stress seem to improve gastrointestinal symptoms, and adding some "healthier" strains of microbes seems to improve psychological symptoms.[300]

- Things that harm our environment like pesticides, cleaning products, and antibiotics, are harmful not just to us but also our intestinal friends, so careful consideration of the absolute necessity of every product we use is essential.

The medical community is thankfully realizing some of this slowly, but as of my time in med school and residency, I had no idea about any of this, except of course that "vegetables were good for me." During residency, when a patient had an autoimmune disease, my only certain goal was to suppress (meaning, make less functional) his or her immune system with chemotherapeutic agents. Infections were treated quickly and fiercely with antibiotics, especially given the patients' depressed and malfunctioning immune systems. Much of the information we have now wasn't available then, but even before this newer detailed information on the microbiome and our immune system, I wondered whether a multi-antibiotic strategy could be harming more than helping certain patients.

I remember in my shared rural practice shortly after residency, many patients I shared with my boss had had chronic or repeated infections over many years, long before my time there. There were adults who were diagnosed with sinusitis a few times per year, children with repeated ear infections, women with multiple UTIs who rarely came in to give a sample of urine. Most of these patients' symptoms were spaced out over enough months that it didn't seem excessive to give antibiotics each time—especially when most didn't call back and felt their symptoms eventually got better with antibiotics.

A few months into practicing there, I started doing extensive chart reviews on these patients when I could. I'd check the dates and types of antibiotics they'd been prescribed, and then ask the patients if they'd taken them all. For patients I knew well who trusted me and vice versa, I started trying a different strategy—which I still use to this day. For simple UTIs, I think about estrogen status and ask about sex and bathroom habits. In healthy patients without fever or history of severe infection, I suggest hydration and phenazopyridine at the same time I call in the prescription, asking the patient to wait on the antibiotic. If their body can clear the infection on its own in 24–48 hours, they don't have a fever, and their pain resolves, they don't need to fill the prescription. When a patient has taken more than one antibiotic in the past year or has other risk factors, I do a culture and ensure the chosen antibiotic is effective and as narrow-spectrum as possible.

For chronic or repeated sinusitis, I recommend a trial of weaning off nasal steroids in favor of herbalized nasal oil. Saline rinses are done before the moisturizing oil for excess mucous. If a patient with chronic sinusitis starts feeling unwell with a virus or allergies, I suggest cutting back on dairy and meat and sweets (and eating more vegetables), emphasize more sleep and rest than usual, and recommend drinking plenty of hot water with ginger or black pepper and honey to keep themselves hydrated and their mucous as thin as possible to reduce the likelihood of bacterial infection.

For children with ear infections it's tougher, since seeing a child in discomfort is difficult to bear, and the smaller passageways make breathing, drinking enough, and getting fluid to drain much harder for little ones. If the tympanic membrane has pus behind it, or if the child has fever or signs of serious illness, there is often no option but antibiotics. For children with repeated infections, tympanostomy tubes (small tubes placed in the ear drum) can be helpful to drain fluid, reducing pain and the frequency and severity of infection, and to help avoid antibiotics. But for less sick children, and parents who understand they could call back for a prescription if the child's condition worsened, starting with warmed ear drops, antihistamine, a humidifier, and pain reliever are often enough to get the child safely over the hump of a viral illness. I also suggest Osteopathic Manipulative Treatment, which can help the eustachian tubes and sinuses drain and reduce the child's number of infections going forward as well.

With viruses in general, even when patients swear antibiotics are needed and have helped before in the exact circumstance, I am firm, reassuring, and suggest home remedy recipes to try first. These simple, sometimes helpful, and always non-harmful remedies such as honey and lemon for simple coughs, saline rinses, and extra sleep, give patients something active and new to do. A note for work gives the needed excuse to rest and practice proper self-care, and allows their immune systems time and sleep to turn the corner. In the rare case patients do eventually require antibiotics, they can call back, answer questions about their new symptoms and fever status, and I am happy to call in a prescription. Maybe 10 percent of patients will to end up with bacterial infections after viruses. Ninety percent of the time or more, bodies just need patience, adequate nutrition, and more sleep.

I need to emphasize here that this is not alternative or complementary or even integrative medicine; this is medicine. This is following current guidelines for antibiotic prescribing while giving patients non-harmful activities that help them feel empowered to help themselves—which might help them recover without ever needing antibiotics. This kind of practice requires patience, trust, and good communication, and makes patients happier in the long run.

Irritable Bowel Syndrome: The Cranky Toddler

Another common complaint I often hear about is IBS. Many patients have experienced no luck with Western medicine and have already gone to various alternative practitioners by the time they find me. Many have been told they had "Candida," or gluten sensitivity, or various food allergies, and were told various diets and supplements were necessary. Probably 30 percent of them had improved symptoms with a sugar-free and/or wheat-free diet, but even among those, many had persistent symptoms. One of my favorite phrases from Dr. Chutkyne's book *The Microbiome Solution* is "yeast paranoia."[301] It seems to have taken firm hold in the alternative medicine community.

It's hard to overstate the ridiculousness of this particular fad diagnosis. It is no more valid than the "alkaline water" craze or that agave is healthier than plain sugar. For most patients, taking an anti-yeast medication does not resolve symptoms any more than a placebo does. If someone truly had an overgrowth of yeast extending to their blood (which many of my patients have been told they do), they would be in the ICU, likely near death. The only patients I have seen who truly have yeast in their blood have severe immune deficiencies, generally from HIV, cancers and their treatments, or other overwhelming infection, and sometimes multiple truly emergency antibiotics.

On the other hand, a propensity to yeast overgrowth in the vagina, esophagus, colon, or on the skin, is much more likely a symptom rather than a cause of out-of-balance gut flora, or dysbiosis, which as we've seen can have many contributing causes. Most doctors are familiar with thrush or vaginal yeast infections appearing after antibiotics, and many actually give a prescription for an anti-yeast medicine along with an antibiotic prescription, to be taken after the course of antibiotics is finished.

But most of the time yeasts (and viruses and a number of types of amoeba and even some parasites) live on and in us without causing harm. Only when our immune system is not working and our bacterial friends are not in helpfully balanced proportions do these potential usurpers overgrow enough to cause problems. Particularly illustrative of this idea is the yeast strain that is helpful as a "probiotic" for treating giardia, even in Crohn's patients,[302] and a type of worm that may help cause remission in Crohn's disease.[303]

We know systemic steroids, antibiotics, and chemotherapy are risk factors for yeast overgrowth among myriad other side effects. But for patients with uncomfortable gastrointestinal symptoms with no direct cause, any extra yeast found is likely simply pointing us in the general direction of dysbiosis. The jumble of symptoms called IBS can present with any number of wildly changing intestinal responses to stress and food, apparent food intolerances and cravings, stronger than usual GI side effects to medications, and painful abdominal distress. Blaming the physiological finding of "leaky gut" may help explain some of the symptoms, but it doesn't actually give us a definitive cause or treatment plan, only a list of possible mechanisms and contributing factors.

Instead, it might help to think of IBS as a combination of a predisposition to higher sensitivity to intestinal discomfort, having an Enteric Nervous System (ENS) that is extra sensitive to stress and microflora changes, and having a disrupted microbiome and intestinal immune system. To treat and improve IBS symptoms, one needs to target many issues involving several systems at once. Start by making sure of your diagnosis (rule out more serious or other treatable problems). Then work on fixing your sleep cycle. Keep a food log for a bit to see if any obvious triggers arise, and try an elimination diet if the food log didn't nail down the main issues. Generally, get adequate exercise and nutrition from food you tolerate, and learn new techniques to manage stress, especially stress from the painful symptoms.

Would More Dirt Help?

Now that we know that a highly diverse microbiome, both inside our guts and outside on our skin, leads to improved health and a better functioning immune system, what do we do? Living "dirtier" sounds like it would help, but it doesn't necessarily work to simply get a pet later in life and hope it will "improve your immune system." Living on a farm or with animals, having siblings, and the "dirty birth" best-case scenarios are mainly effective when they happen from birth through early childhood, when the immune system is more trainable. In some cases, adding more variables to a poorly developed or impaired immune system can lead to worse problems. A case in point was my mother, who developed asthma requiring multiple medications after we got a dog. Unsurprisingly, her asthma completely disappeared after our dog died.

It might be a good first step to know the short list of things that contribute most to continuing immune impairment, and use these as sparingly as possible. Antibiotics are obvious, but also topical steroids, nasal steroids, NSAIDs, PPIs, estrogens, antacid medications, cleansers with parabens and triclosan, and possibly any skin cleanser or moisturizer with preservatives or potentially harmful ingredients (check EWG's "skin deep" database), antiperspirants and most deodorants, hand sanitizers, harsh mouthwashes, and pesticide exposures. Any system-affecting drug or supplement may alter our microbiome in ways we haven't found yet, so it's best to be conservative.

As substitutes for the above, food-grade oils work well for moisturizing and mouthwash, castile soap works for cleansing, herbal nasal oils can be helpful for mild allergies instead of steroids, and a salt crystal can work as a deodorant for many people. There are more economical and environmentally friendly ways to avoid many microbe-killing inputs to your system, so I encourage you to be creative and curious and try different tactics for yourself.

In Summary

Once we shift from actively killing off our microbial friends and stop promoting undesirables from proliferating, how can we encourage more diversity and better function from them? The short answer is that we're not sure. Many things that are associated with microbial health are also associated with overall human and environmental health. From overuse of antibiotics (in both humans and livestock) to using hand sanitizers too often, things meant to keep us safe end up hurting our microbial diversity, just as pesticides end up hurting the soil microbiome as well as bees and other important insects. The effects of indiscriminate extermination harm our nutritional status, our immune systems, and our nervous systems, just as widespread pesticide and synthetic narrow-spectrum fertilizers worsen erosion and runoff and cause pervasive damage to ecosystems. In order to turn the trajectory around, gentle but firm overall action is needed. And like our planetary ecological systems, the best courses of action seem to be the least violent and those that take the entire system into account when developing a treatment plan.

Animals we raise for food should live in environments and situations that are the most natural for them. This prevents them from getting sick and needing so many antibiotics, which create resistance and infiltrate the soil and water. Avoiding purchasing animal products from places that regularly use antibiotics for weight gain and as infection prevention will go a long way to breaking the cycle of creating resistant superbugs.

Instead of relying solely on new genetic and microbial-altering technologies, we can take cues from nature. We can bring ourselves back in contact with more microbial diversity, especially when trying to feed and hold onto our beneficial new friends. Stopping practices that are harmful will allow the microbes that are already living to thrive and communicate better with the rest of our systems.

Next, starting to include practices that might be different from what you are used to is best done gradually and gently, so as not to shock your system. This way you'll be more likely to recognize any effects from the new approaches you've adopted that might mean the practices need to be slowed down or changed. Above all, make sure your sleep is adequate, and stress is managed well (we'll discuss how stress can be managed in chapter 8 and meditation in chapter 9), so that your hormonal and immune systems can be optimally prepared to adapt to new inputs.

While probiotic products taken internally, applied externally instead of soap (think of a horse rolling in dirt[304]), or taken for specific symptoms might be helpful, it is probably easiest to start by incorporating more whole foods into your diet. Added vegetables, and best, vegetables from sustainably farmed, healthy soil should be a priority. This ensures pre-biotic food sources for your healthiest strains of bacteria, fresh, nutritious energy for you, soil bacteria to interact with your immune system, to improve the biodiversity and function of your digestion. It also helps local farmers (or you, if you're gardening for yourself) and builds community self-sufficiency. Eating fermented vegetables may help too, as this can train the immune system and help good bacteria to flourish. It seems reasonable to include some cooked vegetables, some raw, and some fermented foods (yogurt, sauerkraut, miso, vinegars) for nutrient diversity for yourself and your bugs.

Branching out from growing food in your backyard or in a pot in the kitchen, consider composting to add to your garden, or if your city has a program, donate your kitchen scraps. Using compost to grow food is economical and less wasteful, improves and builds soil, and increases the soil's ability to hold moisture so less water runs off and less is needed for irrigation. Incorporating animal contact in your life is helpful also, but as with my mom and our dog, be careful about committing to a pet before you're sure you can take good care of it. Also make sure you won't be allergic. Consider fostering from a shelter first, and adopting only if you are prepared for the responsibility. Volunteering at a local shelter and/or getting to know and help out local farmers are also great ways to build both community and your microbial diversity.

Especially with young children, since we know they are more likely to benefit from exposure to diverse microbes, encourage them to get outside, go camping, play, and explore. If you are like my mother, you might be concerned about illnesses from fresh water streams or dirt, and might have a complete aversion to activities like camping in general. While it's necessary to seek medical attention if your child catches something that becomes an illness, remember that, at least in first world countries where vaccines for most of the worst illnesses are readily available, most exposures are healthy training events for a child's learning immune system. Being exposed to pathogens does not mean those organisms will become pathogenic for every person, and, as we've seen, over-cleanliness does more harm than it helps, in most cases. Find programs and camps for your children that encourage outdoor self-sufficiency and, you never know, it might start to look more appealing to you, too!

In this technological age, we really need to stop thinking of ourselves as cleaner than and separate from our environment. A better analogy is that we are chimeras, composed of many different organisms, working together to be able to exist.[305] Our cells communicate with each other constantly, our tissues and organs talk to each other through fluids and nerves, and our microbial allies are an integral and irreplaceable part of the conversation. There are so many interactions with every single thing we ingest and encounter in our lives that more attention to detail is needed to really take care of our microbiome, since it *is* "us."

7

COMMUNITY MATTERS: FARMERS, FOOD, AND ECONOMICS

Environmentalists and "foodies" alike have been talking about ways to help fix environmental problems by altering our food choices for a good long time. My favorite is bestselling author Michael Pollan, mostly because his science is accurate, but also because he has a sense of humor and is practical with his common-sense suggestions. "Eat food, mostly plants, not too much" is still one of the best summaries of what I've found in my own research and with my patients. Back when I first started synthesizing some of these ideas, it was encouraging to me that my ideas about Sustainable Health already had proponents, even if no one else was calling it that at the time. What seems to be needed now is a more complete connection of this triangle of health, the environment, and growing healthy food. In this chapter, we'll look at how these are connected and how to help people, communities, and the environment thrive by encouraging sustainable farming.

Bros: Integrative Medicine and Sustainable Farming

The arguments comparing conventional farming practices to sustainable ones sound to me just like those comparing conventional medicine to integrative medicine. There is a pervasive modern attachment to answers that come from the newest science, a feeling that new ways are automatically better than old ways of doing things, especially if the new ways seem to work miraculously in the short term. At the same time, there is a reluctance to give up practices that seemed to work miraculously a few decades ago, before better information was available. To keep ourselves at an adaptive advantage, we need to be critical of ideas both new and old, while applying new information very carefully. Some new information may be dramatically helpful, like genetic research and new soil microbial science. But prescribing the newest antibiotic for a likely viral illness is just as harmful to a patient as spraying entire fields with fungicide before planting is to the soil structure and the farmworker doing the spraying. Instead, we can use the newest technology to look ahead, treat problems with more precision, and model better system management.

Impressive analysis is available that can pinpoint which nutrients are abundant or deficient in the soil, and which plants might do best, without having to spend years on trial and error as used to be necessary. But we need to remember that good scientific analysis still doesn't mean the solution is an application of a synthetic version of one or two particular deficient nutrients. Instead, using good scientific results can show us the direction we need to move in to help repair soil problems in the best way, allowing the buildup of healthier soil over time. This longer-term view, with an eye to both prevention and building health, is sustainability—this way we are not limiting ourselves to band aids or emergency medicine.

It's the same idea as with cows and higher instances of

botulism infections: if you don't get rid of the cause of the increased infection rates, which may or may not be related to increased pesticide use, then treating the cows with trace elements or vaccines simply treats the symptoms of the problem and is not sustainable or economical. If soil is depleted because of the conventional farming techniques themselves, spot treating nutrient deficits and pest infestations will not do anything to fix the problem in the long run—and might make it worse. Instead, balanced organic composts, animal droppings and trampling, cover crops, and other sustainable approaches actually rebuild soil and reduce erosion, which in turn reduces toxic runoff.

Sustainable Medicine, which is essentially a version of regenerative agriculture applied to the human body, integrates this type of thinking, proving again that the same concepts of sustainability transfer from the environment to medicine and back again. Allowing nature to heal and being surprised by the speed and efficiency with which it does so has been found to be true in ecosystems as well and is easily applied to farming and animal husbandry. For example, when fishing is stopped, depleted fisheries can bounce back decades faster than projected.[306] And introducing predators back into collapsing ecosystems helps return diversity of plant and animal life, which can go a long way towards remedying problems like erosion and habitat destruction in a few short years.[307]

Since ecosystems are complex, of course there are no simple answers, and no one action will completely fix any issue,[308 309 310 311] especially since climate change and pollution are variables we have less local control over compared to fishing or hunting.[312] But ecological science helps us understand the links between each piece of a particular habitat and allows us to find ways we can make big changes by simply allowing a more natural pattern to re-emerge. Working with complex natural systems rather than against them or trying to fix them piecemeal is more effective and sustainable. It is very possibly the only way we can move forward and improve environmental and human health.

I won't go too deeply into the injustices and environmental damage the current farm subsidies perpetuate, but a few points need to be understood from the beginning of any conversation about farming: 75 percent of subsidies go to the richest 10 percent of farms, and the 2014 version of the farm bill again disguised these payments as "insurance coverage."[313] [314] [315] [316] [317] [318] [319] [320] This means huge subsidies and tax breaks continue to favor massive, monocrop-based agribusinesses, including the billions gained by huge grain traders, suppliers like Monsanto, processed food producers of products like high-fructose corn syrup, and major meat producers like Tyson and Smithfield and Hormel. This type of farming tends to overuse synthetic fertilizers, use more soil-destroying pesticides, involve experimental GMO crops, create poor living conditions for animals that favor high antibiotic use and high mortality rates, and often disregards the health and work conditions farmworkers and factory workers are forced to tolerate.

Smaller farmers do not benefit much from these financial incentives, and the majority of economists on both sides of the political spectrum agree that the subsidies make no sense. Taking the wider view, the policy also hurts poor countries around the globe since there is no way they can compete with our biggest taxpayer-subsidized farmers. Huge companies that use a product like sugar to make candy or other processed foods can move their plants to other countries where they can pay much less for sugar, then sell their products back to us, widening their profit margins, while our farmers are then paid by our government for producing extra sugar and corn at too high a price.[321] [322] [323] [324]

Clearly this type of policy is not a sustainable or globally scalable solution to feeding the exponentially rising population. There is ample research that smaller, more sustainable farming including urban farmers and backyard plots, *is* sustainable, uses less energy and produces less greenhouse gas, and is scalable globally, as explained by the U.N.'s 2016 report.[325] Organic farming yields match conventional yields when compared correctly, sustainable farming outperforms conventional in years of drought, and is more profitable and less energy-intensive than conventional farming over time. One of the most important points when discussing practices that promote long-term sustainability is that sustainable practices build rather than deplete soil organic matter, leading to increased productivity, better water conservation, and improved yields in the future.

GMOs and Pesticides

I should mention GMOs up front also, just to get it out of the way. I am not in the "GMOs are evil" camp, since I don't believe anything is inherently bad—it just depends how we choose to use the tools we create. But genetically modified (GM) seeds that are used in an overwhelming majority of crops in the U.S. create and perpetuate problems that can be alleviated by sustainable farming. GM seeds do not have higher yields, their use creates herbicide-resistant weeds and insects, which require more toxic exposure for farmworkers and soils, and farmers who use GM varieties earn less money.

Widespread use of Bt, a toxin produced by a gene inserted in corn and cotton meant to kill root-eating insect larvae, has led to resistance to the extent that the company that creates these GMO seeds started inserting more genes so the plants will make more toxins since the first one became ineffective. Even the EPA cautioned against this type of resistance and suggested planting non-Bt crops nearby to attract non-resistant beetles. Insect resistance to pesticides, just like with bacterial resistance to antibiotics, leads to either more pesticide use or worsening crop loss, but the companies and most large-scale farmers leashed to them are slow to change strategy to sustainable solutions.[326]

There may be even more insidious problems with GMOs. Bt has been found in human blood, and eating GMO corn can cause immune dysfunction in mice.[327] [328] A combination of GMOs' required pesticides, fertilizers, and other genetic alterations that may affect pollen and the plant oils bees come in contact with are likely to be key contributing causes of "colony collapse disorder" (CCD), severely affecting bee hives around the world. Since these huge companies block outside research, and since lobbyists for the companies push "safety" statements through government agencies so the products can be sold, it's very hard to know for sure what is true about GMOs, which is the best reason for caution. In any case, it isn't helpful or prudent to simply blanket all associated genetic technology with an "evil" label; priorities should be better research and labeling, so participation in the GMO experiment is a choice rather than imposed on us unknowingly.

Pesticides and their safety should also be easier to study, but research control and political intervention by large companies has continued to make pesticide safety controversial and the available research questionable, even after the issues with pesticides like DDT and its eventual ban. Crop applications of a variety of pesticides have been linked to childhood asthma, birth defects, cancers, and neurotoxic effects, especially in babies.[329] [330] [331] Due to extensive use not just for weed control but also to dry out plants for harvest, excessive chemical application has become one of the biggest and best arguments against conventional agriculture.

Glycophosphate, a particularly controversial example, has been implicated in causing more botulinium bacterial infections that have become more prevalent in Europe, as well as possibly causing decreasing bacterial diversity in raw milk.[332] [333] [334] [335] Usually cows' microbiomes protect them from botulism, but if their microbiome diversity is low, they become susceptible to botulism. Other factors are correlated as well, such as trace element deficits, but since drugs given to humans can cause similar deficiencies, it stands to reason that pesticide exposure could cause serious problems. If pesticide exposure reduces bacterial diversity in cows and changes how they absorb nutrients, there is no reason it would not have similar effects in humans. More research should be encouraged, not blocked.

As we talked about in chapter 6, we don't know what pesticides and fungicides might do to our own microbiome, even in small amounts, over many years. A few studies point to possible links between these chemicals and human illness, but due to poorly funded and poorly constructed studies, we aren't absolutely sure.[336] It does seem likely that some can affect fertility.[337] But even the *likelihood* of human danger should make us more cautious, especially when there are also pollinators like bees and bats, soil health, and water contamination to consider. Since many species of bees are responsible for 40 percent of our food supply, anything that harms them harms us.[338] [339]

Personally, I have already participated without my consent in long-term experiments with margarine ("It's healthier than butter!"), antibiotic overuse ("Germs are bad!"), and highly processed foods, and I would rather not participate in another untested group of experiments. Safety should be *proven* within reason before, not after, millions of people have consumed a product for decades. "Can does not equal should" applies even more strongly now that science far outstrips the speed at which nature moves.

The Union of Concerned Scientists and the American Academy of Environmental Medicine have both argued against adoption of GMOs before safety is proven because of the cautionary principle, and because of the serious implications of the small amount of data with adverse outcomes.[340] Entire countries (including most of Europe) have outlawed GMOs for the same reasons, but even having a rational discussion in the

U.S. is difficult with the amount of money and political lobbying involved.

To summarize, although I don't think GMOs or any other science is inherently bad, I do recommend caution. Collectively, we must use clear intelligence to decide which solutions will truly be sustainable and beneficial for both people and the environment without which we cannot be healthy.

Organic Food

How about organic food? Although I approve of the movement away from pesticides and fungicides and towards soil and water protection, for now organic food is pricier, and much of it is grown in nearly as industrial a manner as most conventional produce, so I can't state unequivocally that everyone should only buy organic food. In any case, organic does not always mean sustainable, although it is clearly better for the environment than conventional farming.[341] [342] The USDA generally does a good job of monitoring farms that claim to be organic for truth in advertising, but it isn't 100 percent, especially with large-scale farms that supply chain stores. Adding to the difficulty from a science perspective is that the nutritional difference between organically and conventionally farmed vegetables is not yet significantly and consistently quantifiable, although it may be soon.[343] [344] [345]

But we don't choose food based only on nutritional value anyway: if we did, no one would buy ramen noodle packets or doughnuts. The choices we make are based on our culture, economics, location, availability, and personal preference. I can't change any of the first four, but for the last, I would like to change the argument about organics. If you have the luxury of choice, then rather than looking only at the price in the store, consider the following. If you pick up a strawberry that was conventionally grown in the U.S., it was likely grown in a field that was prepared with fungicides, which causes cancers in farm workers and destroys all the soil microbes necessary to fix nitrogen and rebuild soil in general.[346] [347] [348] [349] It was likely sprayed with pesticides and possibly herbicides, which also causes cancers and neurological and reproductive problems in farm workers, and harms beneficial insects like pollinators.

This conventional strawberry was probably fertilized with synthetic material from non-renewable resources like natural gas and mined phosphorous and potassium, with a narrow nutrient profile that damages soil and causes erosion.[350] It is likely more fertilizer than needed was used in several applications over the growing season. Due to poor soil structure because of the above issues, the extra fertilizer no doubt leached through the soil into local water systems, contributing to potentially deadly low-oxygen conditions in streams, rivers, and the ocean, like the "dead zone" in the Gulf of Mexico.

Conventional farming, including GMO crops that are widely planted in the U.S., increases the use of pesticides and synthetic fertilizers. Conventional GMO farming also discourages crop diversity and seed saving, which causes economic problems over the years and around the globe for farmers, and cripples our adaptability to climate change, resistant pests, and new pest outbreaks.

Organic farming, including the even better techniques of sustainable and regenerative farming, is clearly better for the environment as well as for farmworkers.[351] By using organic rather than synthetic fertilizers, along with techniques to build soil and protect soil-building organisms, it can restore damaged soils, which then hold more water and require less irrigation. By encouraging the use of cover crops, seed saving, and care of the wildlife in and around the soil, it encourages biodiversity and reduces the likelihood of devastating monoculture-induced crop obliteration as occurred in the Irish potato famine. Several studies, including the official UN report, have found that organic farming practices are the best sustainable way to improve economies and feed people across the globe long term.[352] [353] While permaculture at the moment is more scalable for small farmers, because of current subsidy policy that favors large-scale agriculture and punishes small farms, basic sustainable techniques can help every kind of farmer still cut back on runoff and carbon emissions.[354] [355] [356]

There are problems with large-scale organic farming as well. Regulations are imperfect, and any large-scale operation tends to promote monoculture planting as well as decreased diversity of wild organisms. Better options include smaller local farms and regenerative, sustainable local practices that when done piecemeal may not meet every organic certification requirement but are still likely to be a vast improvement over conventional farming. Whatever brands you choose, do a bit of "Googling" to see if they've met minimum or better than minimum standards, or if there are other brands available in your area that might be better.

If you can't buy organic, then eating more fresh, cooked, and pickled vegetables of any kind is still the highest recommendation for preventing and reversing disease. But if you can afford to buy organic, or better than organic, then do. It's better for the soil, the community, and likely for your own health.[357] If possible in either case, purchase vegetables and fruit locally, in season, from a farmer you can speak with. Organic or not, you'll be supporting the local economy much more effectively than through a big chain grocery store, especially if you find farmers who are also interested in improving the soil and local waterways.

Farming for the Future

There really are viable alternatives to industrial-scale agriculture we can adopt that will serve both humans and the planet better in the coming centuries. In most of the world, small family farms are the backbone of food security, and their potential for greater diversity and flexibility combined with good policy is likely our best hope to continue to feed humans without causing so much environmental destruction.[358] Organizations like the Rodale Institute have been doing long-term studies comparing both "conventional" (including GMO crops) and organic agriculture practices, and found most of the arguments for conventional farming and the arguments against organic at least flawed, and at worst entirely untrue.[359] [360] [361] [362] In fact, it seems that when done well, and incorporating solid local environmental studies with farming techniques, sustainable agriculture methods can double global food supply with less environmental impact, especially in areas with the most difficult climates and soil types.[363] [364]

Carbon farming, which focuses on sequestering carbon from the atmosphere to mitigate global warming, has been proven to be helpful and was heavily advocated for at the 2015 and 2016 world climate conferences in Paris. As mentioned in chapter 5, different ways of raising livestock may be able to help capture some of that extra carbon and help restore ecosystems as well, and research is ongoing in various plains ecosystem in the Great Plains of the U.S. as well as in Africa.[365]

Another bonus of sustainable farming practices is that they are inherently adaptable, since the practices are individualized to each climate, soil, and community. Sustainable practices make sure the fields grow diverse types of locally consumable food instead of favoring monoculture commodity crops, which is essential for keeping local people's food secure. These practices encourage seed saving and adaptive breeding techniques, which means local people can perpetuate their own seeds, then use diverse planting and anti-pest planting techniques while fertilizing with compost from their local kitchen scraps and animals. This also means they do not need to repurchase seeds yearly along with synthetic fertilizers and GMO-adapted pesticides. All these adaptive and learnable techniques make for more speedy flexibility when conditions change, which is absolutely necessary with climate change impacts already causing severe long-term droughts in Ethiopia and Somalia, and floods in Bangladesh, India, and elsewhere. Flexibility and quick adaptation is something conventional agriculture cannot provide.

But systematic changes need to be looked at carefully. The marketing of "cage-free" eggs is a good example of this.[366] While chickens are healthiest if allowed to roam and peck bugs from fields ruminants were pastured in the week before, buying eggs with a "cage-free" label doesn't mean that is how the chickens who produce those eggs live. A few major fast food companies have noticed that their customers care how their food animals are treated, and these companies see that the idea of chickens in cages they cannot turn around in sounds terrible, while living "cage-free," sounds like a great idea. But if no other regulations are followed, it might be a worse situation if tens of thousands of birds are allowed to roam freely in an enclosed warehouse with a concrete floor. Chickens are social animals, but when confused or overwhelmed they can behave aggressively. And when thousands of birds wander free in an enclosed space, their waste is much harder to cope with, which endangers both the animals and the farmworkers.

This brings us back to flexibility and good research. The fact that "cage-free" is sometimes arguably worse than tiny cages doesn't mean there aren't alternatives that are safer and more compassionate. It just means that the interim solutions that will take us closer to a truly sustainable farming economy are not black and white. It requires backing up and looking at the issues with a wider lens to come up with economically viable solutions that can make conditions better now and lead to even better future conditions. It also requires that consumers recognize the difference between misleading marketing words like "natural" and "cage-free" versus labels that may include better descriptors of sustainable farming practices, or at the very least, known regulations such as "pastured only" and "certified organic."

Farmer Friends

Knowing your local farmers can get rid of the disconnect many of us have with our food, and by extension our health and our planet. I've bought eggs from a man in a Carhartt jacket who knows all his hens' names. My favorite strawberries came in a paper box from a mother of a toddler who was eating a carrot covered in dirt. I once bought honey from a quiet man in Texas whose three rambunctious daughters in various states of dirt-covered creative dress played happily around his truck bed and gave me tips on what foods to top with their honey. I've planted happy seedlings from a friend who had found and rebuilt a used greenhouse to allow her to grow medicinal herbs as well as to expand her seedling business. These experiences are so different from buying a piece of pale chicken covered in plastic on a Styrofoam tray, or strawberries in a plastic container picked in fields toxic to farmworkers, or anything in a box with a label telling you it will heal whatever ails you.

My encounters with farmers as an adult have widened my understanding of farming and the local economy exponentially. I grew up with a cornfield literally across the street from me, but I wasn't allowed to explore it. My mother may have been afraid I would get lost or bitten by something. She also discouraged me from taking a "detasseling" job, which is essentially controlling the reproduction of genetically modified corn, something many Mid-western kids do to make money each autumn. At the time, I had no idea the fields behind my house were growing corn and soy to feed livestock rather than people. I'm pretty sure my mother had no idea either, and we certainly didn't personally know anyone who farmed, even though they were our neighbors and their fields surrounded my hometown.

The suggestion to get to know who produces your food is strangely revolutionary at this point in our food culture, but in times past it was normal. The "local food movement" would have seemed ridiculous to people 200 years ago, when nearly everyone ate what was grown locally. Then, very few foods would travel well or fast enough to be sold far from where they were grown. But now, in most chain grocery stores, there are noodles and shrimp from Asia, apples and asparagus from South America, cheese from Europe, meat from New Zealand, and spices and grains from the Middle East. Pasteurization, refrigerated planes, food radiation, new packaging technology, and extreme processing all allow food to last weeks to years on shelves, and have expanded export and imports to the point these things are expected. It is difficult to imagine where and how the farmers who produce such things live and what they are like as people. Fortunately, good journalism and great video series like "The Perennial Plate" help us learn more about what it means to farm and produce amazing food, especially sustainably.[367]

But for those of us who live near spectacular farmers' markets like the ones in Santa Barbara, California, or where roadside stands are ubiquitous in the summer, like in Georgia or Texas, knowing farmers from the market can be a normal part of life. If you've never done this, I encourage you to make it a new habit: During your county's growing season, find an available farmers' market, or one of those tiny stands along a highway you pass regularly. Instead of driving by, stop. Talk to whoever is standing there selling their wares. Find out where the farm is and how they take care of their crops or animals. (Asking these sorts of questions can clarify whether they are growing the food themselves or buying flats of produce from a wholesaler and re-selling for local convenience, which happens quite often on the West Coast). If you have time and you like their products, ask if you can visit their farm. When I lived farther out in the country, I had several friends of friends who were farmers, so it was easy to get to know some of those hard-working people who are so passionate about what they do.

Buying groceries locally when you can is most helpful from an environmental standpoint if the farmer takes good care of the local soil, water, air, and farmworkers. It improves the local economy, builds community, and helps ensure local job security. Not every product is best purchased locally however, as several studies have pointed out. Carbon footprints can be worse when people buy difficult to grow or out-of-season produce. For example, tomatoes grown in local greenhouses in northern Europe in January can require more energy for temperature control than would be required to ship from a country slightly to the south. In any case, when you can, buy in season and locally, but if you must buy products from far away places, aim for products with organic and fair trade labels. While not 100 percent reliably ethical, these products are likely to be better for farmers and the environment than the alternatives with no regulation at all.

If you know where your food comes from, you are more likely to know whether the environment and farmers were harmed in its production. Buying from a farm you know means the food will be fresh and possibly picked that morning. Paying farmers directly for the food they produce means they have a better chance of making a living from their work. Strengthening the local economy by ensuring that farming is profitable is a way to ensure food security and strengthen the economy in general.

Paying farmers directly also means you contribute less to large chain grocery companies who pay farmers a low wholesale price and then sell the food to customers at a profit. If you end up paying slightly less for produce at a big store, imagine what the farmer was paid, how far it likely traveled, and what practices may have harmed workers or the environment that go unnoticed by consumers on a daily basis. These invisible costs of big business and big agriculture are still costs; we just all pay them later.[368] [369]

Making good decisions can seem daunting to the point of resignation, especially when problems like pesticide and fertilizer poisoning of farmworkers and economic hardship for farmers are in the news. But very much like we talked about in the last chapter, there are simple things we can focus on, and even a small change in consumption patterns by many people can have wide-ranging positive repercussions. Of course, while this idea of choice only applies to those of us who have the economic power to choose, that still means 70 percent of people in the U.S. have the power to make better food choices, even if only occasionally and in carefully chosen circumstances.

Finding out where your food comes from is also one of the best ways to more fully enjoy and appreciate your food. Although in many areas the growing season is a very brief seasonal event, it is well worth venturing out to explore the farms in your region. Be curious and ask questions, and buy sustainable produce when you can. If you don't have access to farmers markets, there still may be a CSA program near you, or a local store that pays farmers reasonable prices for their produce. And in some states, SNAP benefits can be used for CSA purchases.[370]

Growing Your Own

If you have any interest in growing your own food or gardening in general, go for it. Find local farmers, gardeners, and seed-saving organizations and learn from them. Join a local co-op garden in or near your neighborhood. Ask what grows easily without much intervention in your area and give one or two things a try. Pick plants that either sound interesting or are particularly expensive to buy at a store, like tomatoes or colorful varieties of corn. Worst-case scenario, if nothing grows well, you still may improve your gut microbiome and mood by working with dirt. And, in the best-case scenario, you get to be outside and end up with fresh produce within steps of your kitchen!

For more details about what to grow, what to cook, and how to build community, an approach I like is a combination of the information you'll find in *Blue Zones*, Dr. Daphne Miller's book, and learning what your great-grandmother ate as a teenager.[371] [372] [373] Start by looking at the types of foods you generally enjoy, and see if whole food or more nutritious versions exist. Pay particular attention to your cultural and genetic heritage, as these may help you look back to see what your ancestors ate a few generations back, before processed food was so widely available. For example, a variation on steak and potatoes might be pasture-raised local lamb with cooked fruit and root vegetables with omega-3-rich greens. And a variation on flour burritos with refried beans, rice, and American cheese could be green or blue corn tortillas prepared with corn masa soaked in lime, with *nopales*, black beans, squash, and fresh *pico de gallo* or salsa *verde*.

You can find out about interesting heirloom varieties of plants and animals from local farmers and invite family and friends to try new recipes. You will soon have more food-based community than you imagined possible. Being curious, sharing, talking to famers, and developing experience-based gratitude for your local food community will not only be fun but better for both you and the environment in the long run.

With all this cooking, you will have some food waste, even if you're very good at buying only what you need and use your scraps in soups. A great way to reduce your waste in general is to compost it yourself or donate to a community garden or farm. If you're feeling very ambitious, and have the backyard and the time (and if it's legal in your town), consider keeping chickens (they eat kitchen scraps, are hilarious, and give you free eggs!), goats (they can be rented out to clear fire-prone brush areas, and you can make amazing cheese), or bees (who will pollinate organic fields nearby and plant wildflowers to enrich the local environment and provide honey!). There are classes available in most places that teach cooking, butchering, beekeeping, and gardening, and online classes for those of you in more remote areas. There is always something new to learn and new ways to enrich your plate, your health, and your community.

Of particular interest to me, and something I take as a great sign that the food movement is making serious headway, is the fact that there are many new gardens and farms popping up which help disadvantaged teens, previously incarcerated people, and those with mental health issues by giving them jobs, a purpose, and exposure to nature.[374] [375] [376] [377] [378] [379] [380] [381] [382] Many of these organizations love volunteers, particularly ones that want to learn about urban farming and permaculture, and of course those who are already experts. You can also check out and support restaurants that are educating people about food, farming, and the environment like Blue Hill Farm in New York. Even media like the *Edible Communities* magazine and video series like *Perennial Plate* and *Victory Garden* can spark creative ways you can make a difference in your local community.

Going deeper, find out what food policies are up for a vote in your state, and call or write your representatives and news publications about your views.[383] Farming heavily influences the environment, but it is also a social and economic issue. In addition to improving human health, farming advocates can be huge contributors to positive social justice movements.[384] Playing an active part in connecting yourself and others with nature is extremely rewarding.

Choices and Big Changes

Since our health is inescapably linked to the health of the planet's ecosystems, paying attention to the ecosystems we most directly affect is important. We decide what we eat around three times per day, and those decisions are tied to a number of variables we have the power to affect with our choices. When we educate ourselves on the externalities not included in the price of conventionally grown food, we might be more inclined to value and purchase local sustainably grown food when possible. While it's very true that one individual's choices have little impact on the environment and economy on their own, it's also true that when a large number of individuals choose healthier options, political and economic impacts are felt and changes are implemented by the larger participators in the food system. This is already happening, with increasing numbers of farmers' markets, huge superstores increasing their organic sections, and fast food chains attempting to use more humane animal products.

Bottled beverages are a good example of the power of people making better health decisions over time. The biggest soda companies realized several years ago that sales of high-fructose corn syrup-based beverages were falling as people became aware of the negative health impacts of empty calories. They began investing in fruit-flavored sugary beverages and a bit later started selling bottled tap water as a "healthy" alternative to soda. As of 2015, bottled water made $110 billion dollars a year for the three largest companies, and 30 percent of bottled beverages sold in the U.S. are various brands of water.[385]

Since then, more people have started realizing bottled water is unregulated, most of it is regular tap water anyway, and the amount of plastic used is horrifying from an environmental perspective. This has led to better sales for makers of reusable bottles and home water filters, and over time will hopefully mean we will get even farther away from petroleum-reliant drinking habits. At the same time, more attention is being paid to city water systems, especially after the widespread lead poisoning in Flint, Michigan. The infrastructure problems that lead to higher proportions of impoverished areas being overlooked and ignored occur in every part of the country. In Flint's case, the problem was due to several irresponsible government cost-cutting measures, but was discovered and publicized by a local doctor, Dr. Hanna-Attisha. To improve our public and environmental health, citizen and health professional vigilance and participation is absolutely necessary.

Taxes on sugary beverages enacted in 2014 in Mexico and in Berkeley, California, led to slightly decreased consumption of those zero-nutrition beverages.[386] [387] [388] Since then, other U.S. cities like Philadelphia and Seattle have enacted taxes as well, encouraged by projected estimates of reducing cases of obesity (12,000 cases in 10 years in Philly). A tax in Chicago was short-lived; it didn't raise as much revenue as had been projected and had greater than anticipated public opposition. More data will soon be available, however, since several countries including the U.K., France, Norway, and the U.A.E. have implemented similar taxes. Despite the fact that definitive, long-term data isn't yet available, this type of policy may show that government taxes on unhealthy products can lead to positive changes faster than depending only on education and personal choice to change market direction. The money raised from the taxes can be added back into health programs and education initiatives. There are other specifically targeted policies that may be even more helpful than a tax; some of my personal favorites are increasing SNAP benefits and subsidizing fruits and vegetables.[389]

Like with farm subsidies and innovative farming practices, more research and more individual education is essential for making better choices regarding the food we eat. So much can be done to change our food system and encourage healthier choices, but it requires all of us to pay attention and participate. In an era of powerful marketing by massive corporations and huge amounts of consumer choice, buying anything is a vote. Yes, it's true that one vote rarely makes a difference in economics or politics, and sometimes making decisions that your friends and family don't agree with or that go against the national marketing trends creates conflict. But just like in politics, it's better to think clearly, become fully educated about your choices, and vote with your actions— whether you are at a grocery store, a farm stand in the middle of nowhere, volunteering with a social justice organization near you, or voting on election day. Since government regulation is slow to work and often controlled by money from huge companies, it falls to us—consumers and voters—to consistently make decisions that are better for our health and for the environment. And since companies follow money, as evidenced by the rise of pseudo-health products with labels of "natural" and "healthy," eventually making truly healthy choices can become the "cool" thing to do.

8

STRESS THAT IS GOOD FOR YOU: EXERCISE!

Part of the reason that exercise is so good for us is that, in a strange way, stress on the body makes it stronger. You may have heard the old adage that a broken bone heals more strongly than before, which is actually true. The same goes for many much gentler changes that happen with smaller stresses from regular exercise. Inflammation caused by torn muscle tissue causes muscles to be rebuilt to bear more weight later. Tiny bits of tissue damage from bruising and straining mean that weak points in the body are found out and cleaned up afterwards. Changes in blood pressure and heart muscle beat intensity help the body adapt to stress. Increasing lung capacity during intense exercise improves lymph flow and tissue oxygenation and improves lung capacity at rest afterwards. Although it might sound counterintuitive, "good" stress like exercise makes us more adaptive and efficient at healing, heading off infection, and using energy in general.

Sitting and Your Lymphatic System

One of the biggest contributors to aging and to chronic pain besides smoking is sitting. Somehow, after centuries of mostly being required to walk or ride a horse to get from place to place, in the last 100 years we've transitioned to not only sitting when at home or work, but also on our way absolutely anywhere, even to places less than half a mile away. At this point in history, people spend more time sitting than they do anything else, even sleeping. And if you are like my grandfather in the last few years of his life, much of your sleeping might be done in a chair also.

From a physiological standpoint, this is disastrous. Not only does it slow metabolism dramatically after only 20 to 30 minutes, but the negative effects on metabolism affect both young and old and patients of any health status.[390] Sitting for more than 20 minutes with hips and knees at 90 degrees and the feet down blocks lymph and blood flow up from your lower extremities, and puts pressure on small blood vessels. Over time, this can lead to fluid leaking out of those small vessels, causing swelling in the feet, increased stiffness of the blood vessels in the legs, and contributing to higher blood pressure.

Reduced lymph flow can contribute to infections in the lower extremities and poor wound healing, especially in patients with heart disease or diabetes. Sitting like this shortens your psoas muscles in your hips and back, which affects everything from your legs to your diaphragm. It flexes your lower back and puts pressure on the fronts of your vertebral discs, contributing to ruptured discs and problems like sciatica. It puts pressure on your pelvic floor and weakens your gluteus muscles, and at the same time weakens your abdominal and spinal postural muscles.

Sitting passively shortens your hamstrings and stretches the quadriceps and gluteals. Over time, this tells the stabilizing postural muscles and fascia that "this is the normal resting shape" and makes actively using those muscles more difficult, permanently changing posture for the worse. If you've ever seen someone who's had a stroke or has a neurological problem that causes them to be unable to move a body part, the contractures and weakness that often result, even with moderately good physical therapy, happen for similar reasons. Anything that affects one part of the spine affects the entire spine, which in turn affects the rest of the body, including the internal organs. Sitting and staring at a computer screen strains the neck, the pelvis, and rounds the mid-spine. And since they all interact, the effect is multiplied rather than just cumulative.

Breathing shallowly is normal when resting but becomes more pronounced when one does not speak or move, as when concentrating, especially in a hunched-over, seated position at a desk. Shallow breathing affects muscles in the spine and ribs, and can seriously limit lymphatic flow and intestinal function, partially through diaphragm inaction. Although postural decline is more rapid when combined with osteoporosis (which is also worsened by inactivity), changes to the spine from sitting over time can be dramatic, even without documented bone loss, causing problems with digestion, elimination, breathing, and even swallowing and speaking.

Retirement as Rejuvenation

It's never too late to start reversing these issues, even if you have been sitting most days for decades. My favorite example is a patient of mine whom I met when he was sixty-nine years old. Arthur (not his real name) had a job for years that caused him to lean over concentrating, looking down for hours at a time, and his preferred musical instrument created a sideways-leaning neck posture. In his retired life, he is still extremely busy and active but tends to sit for hours at a computer. When Arthur first came to see me he'd tried numerous body workers, massage techniques, chiropractors, and various exercises, but he felt that in the past few years he'd lost much of his flexibility, agility, and energy, and was concerned that he was speeding toward infirmity. Coming to see me was a bit of a long shot for him, since he'd never had osteopathic work, and I was also new in town at the time.

Arthur is one of the most determined and persistent people I've ever met, and is one of maybe ten patients of mine who has actually implemented almost every single suggestion I've given (I don't even do that with my own doctors!). We were both happy to see that because of his hard work and persistence, his posture improved after just a few visits, with a combination of osteopathic treatment and exercise prescriptions I showed him how to do at home. Over the years, we've worked together to help him with injuries, arthritis, gout, and weight issues, despite unavoidable medical treatment from his specialists that caused weight gain. Like everyone, Arthur has preferences for foods and exercise types that we had to work with, and he also had preconceived notions about both that I needed to discuss with him, giving examples of how he could use his body differently to help correct some of the postural and neurological habit patterns that had developed over the years.

I use Arthur as my favorite example because most doctors, when seeing a patient over 65, would have diagnosed him with arthritis, sent him to physical therapy perhaps, and would have told him to exercise more and improve his diet to lose weight. Those suggestions would have fallen flat with Arthur, as they had before he came to see me. He had arthritis, but it was 75 percent postural, worsened by sitting, worsened by deep tissue massage, and worsened by his occasional too-intense bursts of physical activity.

Before I met him, Arthur already had a healthier diet than 99 percent of people in the U.S., and made a point of exercising far more than average for his age. Physical therapy of the type we worked with was slow, deliberate, changed slightly every other visit or so, and focused on teaching Arthur with his own observable biofeedback. I changed his exercise prescriptions after each osteopathic session, during which I could see him walk and bend and update myself on his progress. We pared back part of his exercise routine and changed other parts as needed. And since he was already nearly vegan, eating mostly whole foods with the addition of fish, his diet was less a problem than for most people. We didn't have access to the individualized genetic and insulin-sensitivity-based testing that is available in some places now, but we saw great progress with his weight and energy levels. After he turned 70, when he received a diagnosis that caused a radical change in his medical needs, we were able to get him through it with maybe a third of the side effects he might have seen without the close monitoring and careful adjustments he was able to make.

Clearly Arthur's case is unusual, his tenacity is unusual, and his drive to learn is above average for a patient of any age. But the best part, and what made the biggest difference for him, was his belief that things could be
better. No matter what medical conditions are present, no matter what age someone is, there is always the chance that there can be less pain, more comfort, better function, more energy, and more strength.

What I've seen work best in practice with all my patients is a combination of concepts:

- First, it is important to counteract habits from sitting, standing, or walking too fast with poor posture with simple exercises, and to break up hours spent sitting.
- Next are common-sense suggestions about sleep, exercise, and food.
- Adding in osteopathic treatment helps break up strain patterns that cause pain and poor posture.
- Making sure to include the latest research in recommendations from a consensus of groups of doctors

helps keep us grounded in good science while being able to tailor treatment plans to each individual.

Exercise at Every Age

Making exercise a priority, especially in the elderly (tai chi in particular), not only prevents falls (and therefore fractures), but it can actually increase brain volume and function.[395] [396] [397] [398] A few years ago, I started teaching my patients something I call "conscious walking." By slowing down their walking movement significantly, patients can play with their gait in order to identify when a joint or muscle hurts, and in which positions. Breathing exercises and yoga poses are other simple exercises that can be done at home and can help locate those areas in the body that are uncomfortable or don't behave as they did years before. This is so valuable—not the nitpicking or focusing on the discomfort—but the identifying of areas that can be improved, and best, HOW to improve them by identifying movements that replicate the discomfort. Being able to bring this information to your physicians or physical therapists is priceless.

There is also research showing that elasticity of brain function improves with exercise.[399] One of my favorite studies used people as their own experiment control by exercising only one leg. It showed that exercise changes the expression of 5,000 genes, which changes energy metabolism, insulin response, and inflammation.[400] Exercise is equal to if not better than antidepressants in some cases, and should be one of the first items, along with circadian-aligned sleep, in a treatment plan for all types of mental illness.[401]

Since infant and child obesity is related to many diseases later in life, children in particular need to be involved in physical activity early on at home and at school, and exercise should be part of a multi-factorial family healthy weight plan. Since technology seems to be the biggest distraction from getting outside in nature, some pediatricians are suggesting banning children from handheld devices until good habits of exercise and creative play are developed, and researchers are now looking at the long-term developmental effects of early screen habits.[402] [403] [404] [405]

Finally, to link back to the microbiome chapter, there isn't enough good research yet to say for sure that exercise improves one's microbiome, but it does make good sense that it would, especially since our gut bacteria are sensitive to changes in our neurotransmitters and mood—which are affected by exercise. I expect the science to catch up soon on this point.

Helpful Ideas for Doctors and other Health Practitioners

Medical teams need to commit to individualizing exercise recommendations and learn how to best achieve the fitness goals that have been set with the patient's participation. This is where research and experience can help, combined with practical ideas that can subtly change how patients perform activities of daily living without having to commit to a gym, expensive equipment, a program, or a specific time of day. A few points are helpful when designing a program to teach medical students, and these same points can help patients understand what they can do themselves before seeing a doctor to provide more helpful information and make their visit most efficient.

1. **Osteopathic Manipulative Treatment** (OMT) or Osteopathic Manipulative Medicine (OMM) is not just "cracking" or "adjusting." It gives osteopathic doctors an excellent advantage and the ability to truly understand how each patient's body is connected. A treatment session can show a physician how posture, habitual movements, and injuries have worked together to create dysfunction. It allows diagnosis and treatment on the table in the office, of course, but best of all, it allows close monitoring of changes over time, and a much clearer understanding of what works and what doesn't for each patient. Osteopathic treatment pays attention to muscle and bone but also fascia, lymphatics, and functional connections during patient movement. These are all important, especially diaphragm movements and connections between neck and ribs during normal breathing. Understanding how these fit together makes an enormous difference in the effectiveness of exercise prescriptions and treatment plans.

2. **Prioritize getting your patients out of the posture they spend most of their time in**. If it's someone who stands all day, get them to sit and stretch on the floor or swim in a pool, and have them walk a few paces with knees up and stretch twice an hour during the day. If it's someone who sits all day, get them up and moving their legs behind them in a lunge twice an hour to stretch their psoas and tone their pelvic floor. For those in wheelchairs and those with physical limitations, simply moving the diaphragm with very deep breathing, doing chair exercises, and prescribing frequent physical

therapy will help lymphatic flow, circulation, and will help prevent problems like pneumonia and issues with continence. The bottom line is that the body is not meant to be stationary in any position for long, and movement is key for keeping the body's systems freely moving and healthy.

3. **Get patients outside**. Outdoor exercise is more beneficial than inside in most cases, and I'm sure the positive research outcomes regarding outdoor exercise will only increase.[391] [392] Just spending a few minutes outside has significant psychological benefits— even a window in a hospital room makes a difference.[393] Exercising outside not only removes one from indoor pathogens and pollutants and stressful associations with work or home, it is also free of charge and allows for a different type of connection that is beneficial in more ways than simple fresh air. There are a number of theories regarding why this is true, but getting adequate vitamin D from sunlight (without sunscreen for 10-20 minutes depending on skin tone, when the UV index is between 3 and 8[394]) and setting a correct circadian hormonal rhythm contribute hugely to health and well-being in ways that a gym cannot. Unless it is actually dangerous to go outside, which does happen, there is never bad weather, only inappropriate clothing!

4. **Encourage your patients to learn about themselves**. Becoming mindfully conscious of behaviors and postures that contribute to pain make them much easier to change. Noting sleep positions, habitual work postures, which leg they stand on when stationary, how they sit to watch a movie or read can all be helpful. In addition, the more information patients can bring you about what causes them pain, what makes it better, and under what circumstances it changes, the better you will be at designing a plan to help them.

Finding Your Routine

If we all agree that exercise is good for us, that it can help overcome physical and psychological obstacles and can connect us mindfully back to nature, how do we choose a routine that works? Let's take the evidence from gentlest benefit to most intense, so that it's easier to know where to start at each person's particular fitness level. A good place to begin is what we've already mentioned: don't sit for too long! Many patients, especially those who are of a healthy weight already, argue that since they exercise and go to the gym many days of the week, sitting can't be an issue for them. The research doesn't agree, however, and from my standpoint, it makes sense that intense exercise doesn't counteract entirely, and certainly doesn't eliminate, the health risks of sitting for too long.[406] Increased risks for specific illnesses from sitting are not dependent on weight or physical ability, and include cardiovascular disease, type 2 diabetes, colon cancer, endometrial cancer, and lung cancer, and these risks increase with each two-hour increase in sitting time.[407] [408]

The risk of death from all causes doubles with long periods of sitting each day, and worsens the more time spent sitting.[409] Several studies prove that breaking up sitting with a few minutes of light walking every half hour improves blood glucose and insulin responses, even during prolonged sitting the following day.[410] In the U.K., this research has been taken so seriously that doctors advise two to four hours of activity *during* the workday.[411] What does this mean? Many will argue that there's no way to spend two to four hours during the day exercising at work, and I totally understand. However, five to fifteen minutes at a time add up quickly, and there are other easy ways to change your position for a minute or two to help counteract the physiological problems associated with sitting.

Taking breaks for physical movement can also be helpful for improving attention and focus, so breaks may actually *improve* your productivity. Make sure to get up from your desk often, even if it is to simply stand behind your chair a bit, go to the restroom, or get a cup of tea or water. Keeping hydrated will help your kidneys and bowels stay healthy, as well as the rest of your systems, and using the restroom more often because you are well hydrated helps prevent infections and things like constipation and kidney stones. The American Diabetes Association recommends three minute-long breaks for movement at least every thirty minutes.[412] If you need a reminder, try using a small timer to help you remember to move your body, whether you stand up, take a short walk, or go up and down a flight of stairs. For times when stepping away from your desk isn't possible, try a few gentle stretches near your desk that help stretch the muscles that become stiff while sitting. This helps break bad posture habits that affect the spine and discs. Pick movements that stretch your legs, pelvis, and back into different positions from the ones they are in when you are seated.

Simply stretching with your arms up, or standing with your heels, shoulders, and the back of your head against a wall for a minute can help correct posture, if you remind yourself to relax your neck and shoulders. If you can leave your desk for two to three minutes, taking a quick break to quickly walk one floor of building stairs once or twice an hour is very beneficial. Adjustable desks are great too, those that can be used as a sitting desk and a standing desk, or ones that can be set over a very slow treadmill. Kneeling chairs and yoga ball chairs can be helpful for posture as well, but they can allow for slouching, so having one or two different chair options to switch between is also a good idea. Changing position is more helpful than a static position period, so any way you can move more frequently during the day will reduce your risk of disease and lengthen the healthy part of your life. This applies to home screen time as well, since sitting watching television or playing video games can be even more passive and metabolism-slowing than interacting at a job.

What About Dedicated Exercise?

Making time for exercise for its own sake is stimulating, controls weight, and can be incredibly fun and rewarding, especially interactive sports like tennis or soccer. Intense yoga and kickboxing were my personal favorite strengthening activities at different times in my life. But, also from experience, injuries sustained from overuse or directly from the activities can take months to years to fully heal, and can completely derail a weight management and strengthening plan. Not to mention that injuring yourself to the point where your favorite activity is impossible is incredibly disheartening.

My personal goal, and the goal I encourage my patients to aim for, especially when you are just starting to increase your exercise tolerance, is to find types of activities that you find enjoyable which you will still be able to do well into your 90s and 100s. Walking is the obvious one here, but tennis, hiking, swimming, yoga, and dance are also frequent favorites amongst my senior patients, even those over 90. The great thing with these types of movement is that you can up the intensity easily and create intervals for yourself if you want to improve your metabolism and/or weight.

Being Overweight: Unfair Stigma—But Real Health Risks

I need to mention at this point that while the exact "number" of someone's weight or BMI isn't that important, the "fat but fit" idea has been thoroughly debunked. Being overweight is strongly correlated with most chronic diseases, including many cancers.[413] In one longitudinal study where 18-year-old males were followed for up to 30 years, fit men had a 41 percent lower mortality risk, and the health benefits decreased with increasing BMI. For those with a BMI above 35 (medically speaking, a BMI of 25 is considered overweight, 30 is obese, 35 is severely obese, and 40 is morbidly obese), there was no advantage from being "fit" (meaning "able to exercise at a high level")—the risks of illness and earlier death from being overweight still held.[414] [415]

That said, it is important to understand that someone who is overweight and has no issues with blood sugar, cholesterol, sleep apnea, etc. *is healthy*. The extra weight is not an illness, even if it does indicate a likely metabolic difficulty that might make problems later on more likely. Most people who are over the "ideal weight" for their height have already tried many things to reduce their weight—they've been dealing with social stigma for years, and they don't need the medical system badgering them further about it. For optimum health, the whole person needs to be addressed, and if lack of exercise, poor eating or sleeping habits, other illnesses or medications, genetic or microbiome factors, financial issues, or life stress are the reasons for the extra weight, these need to be addressed exactly in the same way they are in a patient with a lower BMI, but perhaps with more intentional gentleness. Discrimination, blaming, or shaming will never help someone become healthier.

It is worth knowing that BMI is not very helpful for estimating the health of large-boned humans or athletes, so don't take that number too seriously either. If you are in a grey area, it may be more helpful to have your body fat percentage measured. It can help you know where you stand, and if you're a numbers person, to follow your progress more reliably if you change habits. I use BMI and body fat percentages only as ballparks from which to gauge progress.

The easiest criterion to use that seems to have the best correlation with inflammation and risk for diseases like cancer and diabetes is waist circumference. The numbers are simpler to remember and generally apply to people in the 26–35 BMI range: for men, more than 40 inches, and for women, more than 35 inches. Intra-abdominal fat is more dangerous health risk-wise than subcutaneous fat, so focusing on reducing waist circumference to lower disease risk is much more helpful than general fat percentage or overall weight.

An important note, especially for adults over 65: being *slightly* overweight is protective (10–20 pounds or so). For those patients, being thin is *not* associated with better health. Again, no one should use these numbers as absolutes: just like not everyone metabolizes every calorie the same way, not everyone's weight can be judged by a table or guideline.[416] [417]

The goal of this book is to help everyone head in a healthier direction, not in regard to some number or appearance, but rather to a state of whole health that is less prone to inflammation and disease. The idea of Sustainable Medicine is primarily about prevention and disease reversal, so the concept necessarily meets everyone where they are without judgment and looks at the interconnections that can be harnessed to improve health. This means that while I am 100 percent body positive, and I sincerely believe everyone is perfectly beautiful exactly how they are right now, I can't pretend it's healthy to be overweight. It's not healthiest to leave depression or high blood pressure untreated either. This doesn't devalue or blame anyone, or even assume anyone wants to deal with those issues with me—in my office the first time, or any time they come to see me. It just means that being overweight is a complicated health concern that would best be addressed, but only when the person is ready—just like any other health issue.

As a doctor, I want everyone to live their healthiest life and prioritizing health may include reducing weight, but maybe not in the way people are used to hearing. Exercise improves cardiovascular and immune and brain health. Improving sleep helps balance hormones and metabolism. A healthier diet improves immunity and all body systems, and there is evidence that healthy eating is particularly effective in people who are genetically predisposed to be overweight.[418] Stress management improves mental health, which supports general health. And all of these things may lead to weight loss, but indirectly, so weight doesn't need to be the primary goal of treatment. In my opinion, weight gain is so multifactorial that it is unfair to focus on it as a problem by itself, and instead, we should look at the conditions that are being maintained to support a heavier body that is more prone to illness, and then work on improving those conditions.

Take It Slow, Start Where You Are

If you have not exercised much, you need to ramp up slowly. Let me give you an example from my own life. After my last major injury, I re-injured myself a few times by increasing my exercise intensity too quickly. After seeing many practitioners, about three years out from the initial injury, I gave up since everything I did seemed to hurt. I walked to and from normal life activities, but I didn't exercise and so I lost muscle and energy. And I still had pain from the injury that kept me awake at night.

In the end, I decided I'd rather be able to move if I was going to be in pain anyway, so I started to exercise very slowly. I pretended I was 108, so I would be kinder to myself with fewer expectations, and tried to remember to be as gentle with myself as if I were speaking to my grandfather whom I adored. I started walking very slowly for 10 minutes every day, increasing this by a few minutes each week. I did the "conscious walking" I taught my patients. I took the day off if I had a painful flair, and started walking low hills. I graduated to hiking, and eventually could walk four miles again. Since then I've had a few setbacks, but each time I knew I could return to being very gentle, lower my expectations, slow down, let myself heal, and start again.

So what recommendations are best, and what should people aim for? There is so much information out there, and there are so many people with ideas about how everyone should optimally exercise, it can be confusing to sift through it all. It's good to know that any exercise, even "weekend warrior" spurts of activity, is better than nothing.

First, if you have any concerns, be sure to check with your doctor, especially if you've had injuries. If your primary care doctor isn't an osteopath, it may help to get a referral to one or to a good physical therapist. Either can help you with an evaluation of your exercise capacity and help you design a plan to increase it while rehabilitating or accommodating any injuries present. If your doctor clears you, try the following: If you are just beginning, start by walking half as far as you think you can, then back. Increase the distance slowly but steadily, so you can do it without injury, until you can tolerate increased heart rate and breathing. Keep going slightly faster and gradually incorporate hills until your muscles and joints are stronger and flexible enough to tolerate quicker movements with less risk of harm. See if anyone would like to join you on your walks, since social support is helpful for many people.

When you are ready to try a bit more, keep in mind the following for future goals:

- Running slowly for 5–10 minutes per day helps cut cardiovascular disease risk.[419]
- Climbing stairs a few times a day can help reduce blood pressure, even if your blood pressure is already elevated.[420]
- Moderate physical activity five times per week decreases waist circumference, decreasing inflammation and risk for diabetes and heart disease.
- Vigorous activity improves both waist circumference and glucose tolerance.[421]

A mix of exercises and slight changes to your routine every six weeks helps avoid muscle "laziness," which is how I describe muscles getting "too efficient" at an activity, and what personal trainers sometimes term a progress "plateau."

If you are cleared to try vigorous activity and you want to, let's look at some official recommendations. The Centers for Disease Control (CDC) says that adults need two hours and thirty minutes per week of moderate-intensity exercise (fast walking or slow jogging, ballroom dance, gentle swimming, non-competitive tennis), or one hour and fifteen minutes per week of vigorous activity (competitive soccer or basketball, hiking uphill, racing, running, or intense swimming) plus two days of muscle-strengthening exercise.[422] Since walking can be done in intervals, you can achieve the goal of two hours and thirty minutes using two 15-minute brisk walks five days a week, and go uphill or up stairs to increase the intensity. This small amount of exercise reduces your risk of death by 20 percent.[423]

You might think that more is better, and that is true, to a point. Twice as much time per week reduces mortality risk by 31 percent, and three to five times the recommended minutes reduces mortality risk by 39 percent. Including vigorous activity can increase that benefit up to 54 percent.[424] In adults over 60, doing some exercise, but less than the recommended amount still decreased mortality risk by 22 percent, while doing a bit more reduced it by 35 percent.[425] And although some studies suggest that "super-intense" activity can be harmful in the long run, in cases of marathon runners and triatheletes, those same studies found that simply doing more activity than suggested, up to 10 times the recommended time, wasn't found to cause any harm.

Adding Intervals

To optimize exercise, or perhaps increase effort above baseline for a time in order to reduce weight or increase general fitness, it's important to know that starting with a small effort can lead to big changes. If you're ready to increase your effort, my personal favorite is adding intensity intervals to what you're already doing. This applies whether you're walking, running, biking, or swimming. Here are the basics of how to do this: At whatever speed you usually go, add a few bursts of "faster" or even "sprint" speed during your workout without adding extra time to your usual total time. Begin with two or three intervals of 10-30 seconds during your usual activity to see how it goes. If you feel well, and feel more physical effort (heavier breathing, increased heart rate) without feeling discomfort or shortness of breath, you can add more intervals or go faster during the intervals.

Research confirmed that just three 20-second, extra-intensity intervals during a 10-minute bike session three times a week improved exercise capacity, blood pressure, and muscle metabolism in overweight sedentary patients, and in men, improved blood glucose control.[426] [427] Although that regimen is likely the minimum that will have any health benefit, it's still pretty heartening and definitely doable as a start. In the case of most patients, starting with small expectations and having success is the best recipe for continuing and improving over time.

For those who enjoy a challenge and like doing physical activity, my personal recent favorite is the 30–20–10 interval idea from research at the University of Copenhagen. I'll write instructions in terms of walking and running, but this type of workout can be done on a bike, a rowing machine, or in a pool, and the warm up and faster speeds can be done at any personal fitness level.

Here's how:

1. Start with a few minutes of warm-up (walk or slow jog);
2. then jog for 30 seconds;
3. go a bit faster for 20;
4. then sprint as fast as you can for 10 seconds.
5. Repeat this 5 times;

6. then stand or walk for 2 minutes;
7. then do another set of five 30–20–10 intervals.
8. Cool down for a few minutes.[428]

If you really go all out on this, it improves blood pressure, exercise capacity, and speed dramatically. It is surprisingly fun to do, and you can work up to it (as I had to). You can try it out more slowly by adding 5-minute intervals to your usual walk, walking normally for 30 seconds, quickly for 20 seconds, then jogging for 10 seconds, and only doing one of the two 5-minute interval sets for the first week or two.

Whether doing the walking version or the truly sprinting version, after you're used to it, you can add a third interval workout per week. Make sure to have at least one rest day between interval days. You can also add another set of five-minute intervals after the second set if you're already in excellent condition.

Go Outside!

Through all of this, I would encourage everyone to do most exercise outdoors, as close to nature as you can be depending on where you live. (More about this in chapter 9.) With adequate clothing, most weather is manageable. Consider joining a hiking group or taking a few 10-minute outside walk breaks during the workday instead of smoking or snack breaks. Very simple changes can lead to much bigger health benefits quite quickly, so I encourage everyone to start where they are and enjoy their current level of fitness to the fullest—outside as much as possible.

Beware Pseudoscience and Exercise Gurus

One of the most frustrating physician recommendations I've ever heard came from a study guide for the Integrative Medicine board exam. The doctor had done years of research. He put together what he believes is the optimal exercise program for everyone. But his program is excessively complicated. It involves a specific combination of supplements in a drink that is to be sipped throughout the exercise time, and a rapid and intense circuit of exercises and weight lifting that probably 85 percent of my patients wouldn't be capable of from the start. Many of my patients haven't exercised in a while (or ever, in some cases), and some require wheelchairs or have chronic injuries. Many patients who are athletic, or were in the past, derive joy from the particular activity they participated in, and those patients often just want advice on how to improve their performance.

The second problem was that I didn't actually buy the conclusions from his research. The study wasn't long term, and it emphasized antioxidants. Antioxidants seem to be a good idea in theory, but other research shows that our body actually benefits from the oxidative stress that happens during exercise (and during a fast), so taking antioxidants while exercising might nullify some of our work, or even be counterproductive. Add that to the fact that most supplements don't work like the food equivalents do, and this particular program's logic collapses.

I found this disappointing, given that it was the major advice in a study guide for physicians interested in lifestyle medicine. If even the physicians who are interested in exercise have trouble sifting through the available research, how on earth are patients supposed to? As much as I wanted to rewrite the entire study guide, I let it go and kept doing my own research and working with patients individually. Clearly the jury is still out. The most important recommendation I have is to individualize your program to your needs and your quality of life. Remember to go slowly with new activities and ask for help when you need it. Exercise should be work, and may push the limits of discomfort at times during higher intensity training, but there is no reason for it to be expensive, complicated, and certainly not painful.

Yoga

My personal story might give you incentive to try yoga if you haven't already, and also may help you avoid pitfalls. I started practicing yoga in college, and enjoyed learning the Sanskrit names and theory of energy flow for the poses, as well as the underlying philosophy. I felt like I was learning a secret code that would help me relax and become stronger. I thought it would let me understand how my body and mind could work together better. When my teacher was unavailable, I taught a few classes and learned how to modify poses for different bodies.

My Achilles' heel (as it was for many of my students) was *Śavāsana*, or "corpse pose." At the end of a class, most teachers recommend lying on your back with eyes closed for a few minutes. Many teachers play music, read motivational or relaxing excerpts of books, and some lead guided meditations. It was my "worst" pose. Back and leg and neck and shoulder pains would flare and insist I move, and my thoughts were like the busiest subway station at rush hour. I'd fidget, I'd occasionally cry, I'd get angry. It was unpleasant, but I thought it was something I had to fight with, and I'd eventually "improve." I imagined the goal was to have a silent, calm mind and a relaxed, rejuvenated body. This image of a future "better" me kept me trying to do a "better" corpse pose for over a decade.

Eventually I learned that allowing my mind to be as it was in each moment, instead of fighting or wishing for better, was more conducive to avoiding overwhelm in the silence of that pose. But around the time I was learning to be more at home with my mind, I started pushing my body too far. I took up a more vigorous style of yoga with the intention of improving my strength, but with a weaker core than I was aware of, I ended up with a herniated disc and sciatica. Despite an excellent teacher, it was my lack of awareness of my own body's abilities and limitations that led me to compete with my idea of a "better" self and hurt myself. Whatever practice you choose, remember that yoga (and practices like it), is intended to bring more awareness and gently guide your mind and body towards more health, so if you find yourself competing, in pain, or in a state of emotional overwhelm, it might not be the practice itself. Approach with kindness and curiosity!

Choosing a Practice

Practices like yoga have been studied extensively, and these practices go a long way toward improving health through epigenetic expression.[429][430][431] There are so many types of yoga—not to mention Pilates, Tai Chi, Qi Gong, and various martial arts practices—that encourage mindful movement, it is easy to find a practice that allows you to settle your thoughts and begin to practice more self-awareness and mindfulness.[432]

If physical activities that require focus, such as surfing or rock climbing or even walking in nature, are your thing, try to set aside time most days to practice. To make any physical practice more meditative, try to first aim for a sense of being fully present. See if you can allow thoughts and emotions to roll away like water off of a duck's back without getting "stuck" in your mind. If something keeps coming up, pause and see if you can look at it objectively, and if it isn't intense enough to require you to stop your practice and address it, maybe save it to think about later, outside of your practice. Remember, if something difficult comes up and you'd like to work through it with help, there are many places to go, from counselors and psychiatrists to hotlines and support groups.

When choosing a particular physical practice, make sure you check with your doctor first, and choose an experienced teacher. Many types of yoga and martial arts are excellent for young athletes, but some teachers may not be prepared to modify or slow down for those who are beginners or have injuries. If your main initial goal is to become more flexible or stronger, start at a level just below where you think you might be and work slowly. The value of mindfulness practices is not in pushing yourself to pain or extremes, but rather in accepting where you are and working with that.

Ashtanga yoga and Iyengar yoga are two of the oldest modern branches of yoga, but are very different. For those of you with boundless energy who need an intense and fast-paced physical practice (each pose is held for one deep breath), Ashtanga may be for you, especially if you are in excellent physical shape. As a caveat, one of my worst injuries came after practicing daily for a year, despite my long previous yoga experience, so though the practice has great potential benefits, one needs to be vigilant and not overdo.

> Bikram yoga is not associated with branches of either of these main types and is mostly a for-profit machine for its controversial leader. If you enjoy it, proceed with extreme caution.

Iyengar, on the other hand—if you find a good teacher—is great for most people looking to start a practice of yoga. It is based on alignment and, typically, certified teachers have spent many hours on anatomy and learning to modify poses for injuries and many kinds of disabilities. Poses are held for longer periods of time and attention is paid more to the "edge," or where tension begins to be felt when actively using muscles, which can be effective in preventing injury from the practice. Another caveat: if you are already extremely flexible, stretching ligaments can make joints less stable, so be careful, even with slower practices.

Kundalini yoga is a more spiritually based traditional practice, focusing on breathing and feeling energy flowing in the body. Many poses and series within Kundalini can be very powerful, so having a good teacher is key here as well. It claims to stimulate the endocrine system, and although no research proves this, my experience causes me to advise caution with some of the more intense and multi-day practices, especially if you are extra sensitive.

With any type of yoga, I would look for a teacher with several years of experience and more than the typical "200-hour" training that most mainstream studios consider sufficient when they hire teachers. There are also a great many low-cost and even free-of-charge options on the internet. I suggest finding a teacher first, if you are new to yoga, in order to learn the basics and have help adjusting for any injuries or anatomical quirks that might come to light. Always be careful when learning at home on your own, and keep your expectations realistic. Like most mindfulness practices, yoga's benefits can be seen right away, but the deepest and most lasting changes are subtle at first and arrive over long periods of time—slow and steady practice is the key.

9

MEDITATION AND THE
HEALING POWER OF NATURE

Meditation, time in nature, prayer, and gentle physical movement are all timeless ways of improving one's mental state and are now proven to have physical and community benefits. There is very good science to support ancient practices like meditation, but when I was in medical school, I don't remember it being mentioned once, although I myself taught yoga for free to students and staff. As studies on stress and modern lifestyle find that humans are unhappy, despite advances in technology and reductions in poverty, other studies are finding that simple daily practices to reconnect with self and nature are cost-free ways to improve our lives, and by association, the lives of those around us. New information shows that meditation can rebuild brain volume, reduce stress, improve sleep, alter gene expression positively, improve immune function, and may even contribute to improved survival in cancer patients.

A great 2007 TIME article was one of the first mainstream acknowledgments that science can now back up—with concrete evidence—what practitioners and teachers have known for millennia.[433] It also pointed out that even psychological practices like cognitive behavioral therapy (CBT) are a type of mindful self-awareness practice and produce more helpful brain changes than medications alone. The study they talk about, which was done on Buddhist monks, is one of my favorites because it very simply connects the regular practice of compassion for others with personal happiness—with brain scan changes to prove it.

In the last fifteen years, substantial proof of meditation's health benefits has emerged:

- As mentioned in chapter 4, meditation can increase melatonin levels and help improve sleep.[434] [435] [436]
- It alters immune and brain function and seems to reduce colds and flus during flu season.[437] [438] [439]
- In prostate cancer patients, combined with lifestyle and diet changes, meditation may be helpful in positively altering gene expression.[440]
- In breast cancer survivors, mindfulness meditation appears to help maintain telomere length, protecting DNA from damage, and correlates with longer survival.[441] [442]
- New research on epigenetics shows just how pervasively helpful meditation can be to health: even a 15-minute practice can change gene expression for energy metabolism, mitochondrial function, insulin secretion, telomere maintenance, and inflammatory and stress-response pathways.[443]

Although most research shows the best results in the most experienced practitioners, as we might expect, it still shows significant and dramatic improvements in many health markers as soon as someone starts a practice. There's no reason to force yourself into a type of practice that doesn't appeal to you either, as even short walks in nature and movement practices can be beneficial by invoking the relaxation response, which is one of the body's best healing mechanisms.[444] Simply taking a break at lunch to experience a garden or tree-lined street can improve focus, lower blood pressure, and create feelings of well-being that increase productivity and improve relationships. Going away from a city entirely and out to a national park or wildlife refuge can be hugely beneficial for work teams and families. Spending a few nights camping can reset the entire circadian rhythm, and the benefits on our psyche of extended time in nature go beyond just improving our sleep patterns.

A meditation practice can be many things, from quick and refreshing to deep and illuminating, and there are enough different types of meditation that everyone should be able to find one that works well for them. Anyone can benefit—even by starting with a few deep breaths on a break outside during your workday. The key is to have a clear understanding of what you are willing to try, what your expectations are, and to communicate with your meditation instructor to ensure you are informed about the technique you choose to begin with.

How I Started Practicing Meditation

After years of practicing and teaching different types of yoga, trying out meditation techniques I read about in books and on the internet, and suffering a number of yoga-related injuries, one sunny afternoon I found myself sitting in a small office in a gloomy building. Across from me, with his eyes shut, was a very thin Ayurvedic doctor who was humming a sound. He asked me to sing it with him. I simultaneously thought I was humoring him, was worried about getting the note correct, and was wondering what made me think it was a good idea to try this. He was my first "real" meditation teacher and part of me was sure I was grasping at straws, but I wasn't having much luck so far with my health issues using Western medicine or the myriad other complementary practices I'd tried, so I thought I'd give Ayurveda a shot.

One of his first recommendations was that I learn to meditate, which he taught free of charge. I was comfortable with the idea, but didn't think I had the patience to meditate on my own since I'd had such a hard time with the corpse pose and brief flirtations with candle gazing and mantra chanting. Still, since I was able to at least attempt those techniques, I decided I would try his for a month or two. He suggested it might take more than six months for me to see benefits, as I had only recently finished residency and had been through some stressful life changes during the same time. I agreed with his assessment of my nervous system being strained, so I didn't argue and decided to take up what I perceived as a simple perseverance challenge. I had no idea how hard it would be for me or where the practice would lead.

In the first three months, what I remember most was the unpleasantness of trying to sit still for 20 minutes at a time, twice a day. My legs and back hurt, my neck seized up frequently, and I sometimes found it hard to breathe. I seemed to get angry every time I tried to sit still, and sometimes found myself in tears, yelling frustrations inside my head. It wasn't until I re-read my meditation journal around six months into the practice that I started to see patterns in the painful thoughts that kept coming up. I realized it wasn't the physical discomfort of sitting that was difficult, but being with the thoughts in my head. Not having a way to distract myself from them seemed like torture. With nothing to look at, no internet to entertain me, no person to direct my thoughts towards, I was truly alone with myself. It took a few more months before the ratio of my meditation sessions changed to being mostly calm and rejuvenating instead of mostly difficult.

In retrospect, a teacher who could have helped me deal with what was happening would have made it easier for me. As it was, the teacher I had simply told me to keep going. In my case, that was adequate, since I had plenty of stubbornness to push through the discomfort—much like how I dealt with medical school and residency. For me, it seemed that learning "the hard way" was something I was familiar with and expected. But like many of my meditation students since then, I found myself often overwhelmed by negative patterns of thought and behavior. Many of them stemmed from childhood, of course, but those were added to the trauma of medical school and residency, and rebounded off of terrible relationships and personal tragedies I had experienced in the years before I tried to learn to meditate. If I had experienced any more difficulties, I might have quit entirely without someone to guide me.

Once my practice smoothed out, it still took a few years to work through the worst of the psychological reasons for how I was reacting. Learning how to simply allow myself to feel or think about whatever arose was actually the hardest issue for me. I tried different techniques over the years: attending a 10-day silent retreat to learn Vipassana, participating in a 40-day Kundalini practice, learning siddhi techniques from a TM teacher I met by chance, taking classes in Qi Gong and Tai Chi, and learning a few other techniques from friends who taught from various esoteric philosophies. In each case I was always looking to find something beyond myself that would fix what I thought was wrong with me. I wanted results, and I expected to become "better" eventually—if I just practiced hard enough or found the "right" technique. I did see results over time—they were just different from what I had anticipated. Improved self-awareness and better control over reactions to emotions and thoughts were the things I expected to happen, but self-compassion was what I was actually learning.

The latest teacher I've worked with teaches a different approach, where you don't try to "distract yourself with this mantra or that procedure," nor does the approach have an esoteric aim or religious philosophy. Instead, the method is essentially about developing tolerance to being with yourself, while being curious about thoughts and reactions and emotions that arise. Sometimes this leads to uncomfortable realizations, but fortunately the method has ways to get through difficulties while teaching you to be compassionately accepting of all possible information about yourself. Becoming more aware eventually leads to being more skillful around one's behavior choices, which is invaluable. I had noticed on my own that this attitude was important and, oddly enough, had started teaching the same concepts to my meditation students—I just hadn't been using them relative to myself very well, until I learned the technique I practice now.

After quite some time, I finally started to become familiar with my thought patterns, my emotional connections to them, and my physical responses and triggers. As more time passed, I noticed there weren't many *new* thoughts, emotional upwellings, or physical discomforts. It was all old news and thoughts I'd heard before. They became familiar, even if the majority were unasked for and disliked by my judging mind—and those were thoughts I recognized also! I noticed there isn't a way to get rid of them, to quiet them, or to change them in the moment, and you can bet I tried everything; at first there is only becoming more tolerant of them, more able to allow them to exist. What was most interesting was the less reaction I had to the unpleasant bits of myself, and the less I tried to make them disappear, the more I saw them as familiar and almost friendly, and the quieter they became. This applied to all kinds of things that came up in meditation: positive, negative, and neutral thoughts, emotions, and physical sensations.

Because of my own experience, and because of the teachers I've had, I've come to believe that beyond the various positive health benefits like longevity, mental acuity, and increased overall life satisfaction—even in very ill patients—the reason to pick up a meditative practice is compassion. If the objective of lowering your blood pressure gets you to try TM, that is wonderful. If wanting to feel better or lose a dress size prompts you to take a yoga class, that is excellent. If fear of aging and brain deterioration or wanting to cope better with a cancer diagnosis causes you to enroll in an MBSR program, I'm thrilled. But in my experience so far, the best side effect of a regular meditation practice is compassion.

The reason this is so important is that when any of us develops more compassion for ourselves, it leaks into the rest of our lives and into our interactions with others. It allows us more time before we automatically react to what happens to us, to others, in the news, or in the world. When automatic reactions are slowed down, we are more likely to be able to respond in a helpful way to whatever is happening. We might even be less likely to react in a way that harms us or our relationships. This means different things to each person, but if you can pause before saying something in anger or fear or judgment, it is much more likely your responses will be better after considering for a moment, and your ability to navigate difficult situations will improve over time.

Meditation is one of those things that will likely improve your life, but might work less well if you have concrete expectations. The relaxation response and health benefits from meditation happen if allowed, but sometimes our brains get in the way and block our ability to relax even while practicing relaxation! The benefits come with consistent practice over time, and are not always obvious at first. No matter what outcomes arise, the side effects of meditation are great, and sometimes the health benefits and psychological improvements can be dramatic. What I've seen to be consistently true for everyone is this: it is beneficial to take a few minutes a day to be silent, and to purposefully set aside time to take care of yourself, to breathe, and to accept how life is at that moment.

It doesn't matter greatly what type of meditation you choose; I'll give examples in a moment. It doesn't matter how long you do it or where you are. If you have kids and have 60 seconds in a bathroom with the door shut, or can remember to breathe deeply at a stoplight on your way to work, or you take five minutes to sit before you pass out after the children are in bed, that is perfect. If you have no interest in sitting or a structured practice, but when you surf you feel a connection to the ocean and the earth and can let go of daily worries and habitual thoughts, you can make that your regular practice. And if you're an overachiever and want to race for enlightenment by meditating a lot in a specific tradition, go for it. But know that this isn't actually a race, and there's nothing wrong with you, so do what you do for the love of it, not out of obligation or expectation of result.

A Student Example

I've taught many students over the years, and while not all of them continued practicing with the techniques I gave them, most have continued practicing meditation in some form, and some have even reached out to tell me how it has benefited them. One of my students surprised me; about a year after I'd taught her my initial techniques, she came to one of my monthly public park meditation gatherings. After the meditation, we chatted a while, and she mentioned how grateful she was that she'd learned meditation and continued to practice it. Apparently she'd been in a job and a relationship that weren't serving her, but she'd been too anxious to see any other possibilities for her life.

After a few months of practice, her partner started becoming irritated at her, seemingly for taking better care of herself and knowing her own mind more solidly. After a few more months of practice, she admitted to herself that the person didn't share her values or support her, so she decided to break off the relationship. Around the same time, she noticed she had stayed in a job she disliked, mostly out of feeling too inadequate to apply for a different type of work that might suit her better. She applied for and got a new position and quit her old job. I hadn't counseled her on any of this directly, but she ended up saying I'd helped her shift her view by teaching her to practice self-compassion. It was lovely to see that she seemed much happier than I'd ever seen her, and that she felt her life choices were more confident and aligned with her true self.

My favorite part of this student example is that the changes I usually see with people who practice meditation regularly are subtle and gentle, and they come from within. Learning to know yourself, tolerate all aspects of yourself (even the negative ones we all have!), and to be more compassionate towards yourself will almost inevitably lead to being more compassionate toward others and being of better service in your life. If it also leads to better blood pressure and an enhanced immune system: bonus!

Some Solid Meditation Techniques to Try

As far as meditation traditions, there are so many floating around it can be overwhelming to think about. The most common type studied and prescribed by doctors is called Mindfulness-Based Stress Reduction (MBSR), established by Jon Kabat-Zinn. Many of the studies done on meditation practitioners using his techniques are some of the best designed to date, and have some of the best clinically relevant results. The beauty of this 8-week program is in its inclusiveness. Many different types of practices are introduced during the program, none of which require a particular belief system, and none of which conflict with any existing belief system. During the last week, participants are guided through creating their home practice, based on what they learned during the previous seven weeks.

MBSR is helpful in treatment programs for addiction, cancer treatment, anxiety and depression, bipolar disorder, insomnia, autoimmune diseases, and chronic pain conditions. It has been studied in schools and improves children's academic performance while reducing violence and improving classroom behavior.[445] [446] It changes the structure of the brain and improves brain mass—even in older practitioners and even with only a few weeks of practice.[447] Mindfulness practices also astoundingly down-regulate inflammatory gene expression in only *one day* of practice.[448]

The 8-week MBSR program can be found free online where you can do it at your own pace. This is a good place to start for anyone who would like to find a twenty- to thirty-minute daily practice, and it has very good scientific backing as far as health benefits go. It also allows you to experience different teachers and to practice different types of mindful behavior, so after the eight weeks you can see which practices worked best for you that you would like to continue, and you can let go of the practices you didn't favor. In-person teachers can be found with a local Google search and are generally very calm and helpful. For those of you who have had a practice before but perhaps are in need of something different, the online teacherless version is a great course.

Another of the most often-studied types of organized meditation is Transcendental Meditation (TM), but it requires a large monetary investment. I would guard against any teacher that says his or hers is the "best way" or the "only proven method" for obtaining whatever benefits you are hoping for. That is never true, and ends up sounding religious, which, if that is not your goal, means that particular tradition is probably not a type of meditation you will be happy with long term.

Other older organized meditation traditions exist, and especially in California, meditation centers and teachers abound. Zen, Taoist, and other types of Buddhist teaching centers are fairly common, and although more austere in their traditions, are ancient and proven techniques. Vipassana has a few offshoots, and although rigorous (the Goenka method requires a 10-day silent retreat your first time), many people find it worthwhile. Recollective Awareness Meditation uses psychology interspersed within a solid Buddhist teaching tradition, and teaches students to meditate with what arises during each sitting.

Many of these types of meditations also add the Eastern practice of serving vegetarian food, in smaller amounts than usual, during the retreats and teaching weeks. Intermittent fasting may be helpful in resetting metabolism and reducing inflammation and insulin resistance, so combining this type of gentle, lower calorie, highly nutritious diet with meditation can be transformative for both body and mind. Often these traditions encourage doing this type of retreat at least once a year, if not seasonally, and serve breakfast and lunch but only fruit or herbal tea for the evening meal. Personally, I find this structure uplifting and much easier than doing it on my own. Rather than feeling deprived, the retreats I have attended with this type of framework have been transformative and enjoyable. It definitely depends on your intentions and expectations, however, and I wouldn't suggest starting with a highly structured silent retreat if you've not meditated silently on your own before.

If you are religious, and want a practice that fits closely with your beliefs, most organized religions have a type of meditation associated with them. Christianity has a long tradition of meditation and mysticism (Thomas Merton, St. Teresa, St. John of the Cross, Hesychasm), although the current preferred term in most U.S. churches seems to be Contemplative Prayer. Meditation is also integral to many sects in Judaism. For Muslims, Sufis, Jains, Sikhs, and people of the Baha'i faith, prayerful meditation is a foundational practice.

Since studies on medical students and residents show that up to *half* have depression symptoms, it seems to me that meditation is one of the best tested and proven ways to help doctors deal with the extreme stress of their jobs.[449] It might be something that, if taught and encouraged culturally in medical schools for stress management, physicians would be excited to teach their patients. Teaching medical students to meditate is a simple and wonderful place to start to turn around the health trajectory of the Western world.

For some of you, a regular meditation practice of any kind may seem impossible. Nervousness, frustration, apparent lack of time, or disbelief that you are capable of sitting still may have gotten in the way of trying any type of mindful practice until now. But there is no rush or "should" about starting a practice. At the same time, the best time to start is always now. Benefits from a meditation practice will be more difficult to come by if your practice is forced, and attempting to cultivate discipline and willpower by "making" yourself do it might work for a short time (maybe even time enough to feel benefits!), but the process, even if successful in the long run, is more likely to be uncomfortable that way. If a scheduled practice seems too much to consider, try a few simple ways to bring mindfulness into your daily life instead.

- For instance, while driving, at stoplights take slow deep breaths, 10 seconds in and 10 seconds out.
- If you become annoyed at someone while driving, at work, or in a store, try to remember the last time you behaved that way and imagine a similar story for the person in question.
- When exercising, for a few minutes at a time, make each step and movement deliberate, breathe more slowly through your nose, and feel your body's energy and vitality, even if simply taking a quiet stroll.
- If you feel stressed during the day, take a few seconds and pay attention to your breathing, to see if you are filling your lungs or not. If you feel like it, take some slow deep breaths, then relax and watch your automatic breathing again.
- When you feel uncomfortable about thoughts or emotions you are experiencing in daily life, see if you can mentally step aside slightly, and simply acknowledge your experience. Cultivating an interest or curiosity in your own reactions can be extremely helpful in changing unwanted behavior and can help generate feelings of compassion towards yourself and others, no matter what is happening.
- Technology can be helpful in several ways as well. Online and in app stores, there are a number of interesting

meditation programs and videos that may appeal to you. Insight Timer is one of my favorites because it has a huge community and can be used as a simple timer, a global social media site, or a place to find a teacher you enjoy. You can see how many people are meditating with you, and it has messaging capability and interest groups. The simple timer has choices for bell sounds if you have your own practice, or you can choose from a number of guided meditations from many excellent teachers. There are other popular meditation apps as well, such as Headspace or Calm, and several binaural beat audio recordings seem safe to try if a traditional practice doesn't appeal.

Since most practices take some time to become routine, changes can be subtle or difficult to notice day to day. Whether you've decided to try taking deep breaths a few times a day, started going to a yoga class, or committed to sitting still with a structured practice daily, keeping a journal can be helpful. Find a notebook with a cover that makes you smile or feel peaceful, and leave it near your usual practice spot. After each meditation or class, no matter how short, make a note with the time and date. If you notice something you'd like to write in detail, go ahead. But after you write, put it away. Not too often, but after several weeks or months, review your journal on your own or with your teacher. Over months and years, differences will become apparent, and changes will become evident around how you meditate and how each session goes. Most interesting, at least for me, is to note how your awareness is changing over time, in your own words, and how the ways in which you react to what arises in your life evolve along with your practice.

If you find yourself eager to quit within days or weeks, please remember my story from earlier in this chapter. Sometimes we can't see the defense mechanisms and habit patterns that have built up, and sometimes meditation, counseling, exercise, or learning anything new can bring them up and into glaring focus for us. So if you pick a practice with a good history and research results, and find an experienced teacher, give it a serious try before giving it up. My suggestion is to stick with a practice, bringing any concerns to your teacher, for at least three but more likely six to twelve months before re-evaluating. If it isn't enjoyable at that point, and if you can't find anything that makes it seem worthwhile, then yes, try a new type, but give the new type a good long chance as well.

Just like any other health practice, diet change, or exercise type, miraculous, immediate results are unlikely and can actually be dangerous. As neuroscientist Mark Mattson said about trying his intermittent fasting diet, you wouldn't try to run a marathon the first time you ever tried running, and you certainly wouldn't expect to be fast. In the same way, you can't expect to find "Zen" the very first week you manage to sit daily, and you can't expect your blood pressure to be better outside meditation that first week either.

Another thing to keep in mind is that meditation isn't something that can or even should remain static and inflexible over time. One of the reasons to meditate includes allowing what is, without expectations or judgments. While a regular practice, even a short one, is most helpful at first, throughout your life different practices may become more appropriate than the first one you went with. My favorite quote regarding this is by Natalie Goldberg, a writer and Zen Buddhist: "There might be periods—a year or even two—when we can't get to the cushion, but that doesn't mean we give up. This might be the fourth rule: We can still carry meditation inside, still see and feel as a meditator, but physically practice differently."[450]

Whatever practice you choose, I encourage you to cultivate curiosity. Curiosity is the opposite of hard assumptions that lead to judgment. You can cultivate curiosity about your practice, how it affects you, what thoughts come up, what associations occur to you, and what physical and emotional changes you notice. Being curious helps you deal with anything that arises in your practice with child-like interest, rather than habitual or negative dismissal or judgment. Remaining curious about your own reactions during your meditation practice helps you develop a better sense of humor about yourself, about your interactions with others, and about the behavior of others as well. Cultivating curiosity helps foster compassion, even if that isn't the intention of your practice per se, and nurturing friendliness towards yourself is a major help in being friendlier to others. As far as sustainability is concerned, being curious, compassionate, and friendly toward ourselves and others is the only way we will collectively be able to understand each other and make the world more inclusive, equitable, and peaceful.

Over the years, I have been through several meditation training classes and retreats, all of them after my residency. The beauty and effectiveness of the many different types of practices is astonishing to me. As I began to teach patients and students to meditate, I was humbled by the changes some were able to make due to their new perspectives on life brought about by a simple, non-religious, self-tolerance-based sitting practice. Nothing I have done has improved my life more (and allowed me to change for the better) than keeping a curious and open mind and working consistently at becoming more aware of myself and how I interact with life. I highly recommend embarking on such a quest yourself.

The Power of Nature to Heal Our Technology-driven World

Let's start with *vis medicatrix naturae*, the idea that nature evokes an internal healing response. Since the 1990s, the field of ecopsychology, or environmental psychology, and more recently the practical application sometimes referred to as ecotherapy, has been studying and working with the beneficial results on human behavior and health from interactions with nature.[451 452 453 454 455] Some scientists in a field called physiological anthropology are working on finding out how exactly nature influences our physiology, even looking at whether there are molecules in the air around trees that are good for our nervous systems.[456] There is also plenty of evidence of the opposite effect our technology is having on us, wherein our increasing dependence on screens can be detrimental to our health, particularly for children with their more vulnerable and still-developing brains.[457 458 459 460 461 462]

I have a relatively new patient I'll call Carl, who has been a diabetic for 30 years and has constant trouble with sleep. The other day we were talking about his blood sugars, and I also asked him about his sleep routine. It turned out he'd "tried everything," and was currently trying to wean himself off one of the most powerful sleep drugs commonly prescribed. After a brief discussion of how the drug works and how his sleep structure might be affected after many years on the medication, he seemed nervous that his sleep might never be better without medicine. I asked if he ever went camping. It must have seemed like a silly question, because he smiled when he said "yes," and cocked his head to one side quizzically. I asked how he slept after a day or two out in nature, without electronics. His eyes got wide and he said, "Fine! I go to sleep earlier, wake up earlier, and sleep much better." So I suggested he take a few camping weekends while weaning off the medicine to help his body adjust back to its own circadian rhythm. I'm confident that when I see him again, the news will be good, and his blood sugars may be steadier to boot!

Children and Technology: Be Extra Careful With Growing Brains

Official recommendations are that children under and up to one year old (and I would say up to two years old, for sure) should not have access to handheld devices or video games, and limiting their television time to an educational 30 minutes (or less) per day is best. It likely depends on the child, but for children between two and eight years old, less than an hour a day seems prudent, and encouraging creative and outdoor activities would be helpful for the entire family. Limiting passive television and screen time (including handhelds) for children eight to twelve years old to two hours a day is appropriate.

Recent studies have shown that reading aloud a physical book instead of an e-book (even an e-book with interactive features) improved interaction between reader and child, allowed more time for questions from the child, and involved far fewer negative interactions, such as "Don't touch that!" during the story. Video games and internet use are a peculiar issue since they can be educational, or even necessary, for homework, but including that time in the two hours total per day and adding improved nutrition, time outside, and adequate exercise would make these recommendations much more well-rounded.

Aside from just saying "no" more often to screens, pro-active developmentally beneficial activities are even better. These types of activities create positive feedback from a brain chemical perspective, just like the dopamine reward pathways video games and social media prey upon. Meditation is also increasingly proven to improve self-calming and compassion, to decrease reactive behavior, and to reduce school violence in school-age children. The more children are taught to have a regular meditative practice, and the more they are encouraged to spend time outside, the better their school performance will be, and the more socially and emotionally adept they will become.

Activities involving in-person social contact outside of school with age-mates are necessary to help children develop social skills. There is no online equivalent for unconscious facial expressions, posture, or variations in tone of voice. Communicating by text or instant message the majority of the time teaches kids that when an interaction becomes uncomfortable, they can walk away from the screen and make an excuse later. If they behave cruelly, they don't witness the other child's facial expression or tears, which distances them further from responsibility for their actions. Early technology-based relationships teach adolescents that the best way to handle emotion or social awkwardness is to take time to hide their reactions and craft a witty or nonchalant response. But social awkwardness is actually valuable for learning how to interact as fully functioning adult members of society, since even negative interactions can teach children about their own responses and emotional makeup, assisting in growing self-awareness and compassion for self and others.

Spending time with family, and parents in particular, on a regular and scheduled basis, teaches children that parents are present and available and that family time is required and important. Further, spending more time with their children means parents are more likely to be alerted earlier to possible dangerous or negative behavior patterns, which may allow them time to intervene before serious consequences occur. Especially for high-risk children and families in difficult economic circumstances, time with trusted adults is key for keeping kids in school and out of trouble. Having dependable role models to spend time with, who are good behavioral examples, can be a step in overcoming hardship, family troubles, and risky behaviors. There are great programs available like Big Brothers/Big Sisters and Boys and Girls Clubs, and when possible, time with a reliable parent that is scheduled and emphasized can go a long way to give a child a sense of stability, no matter what might be happening at home or school.

Combining social time with outdoor time—and even spending alone time outdoors—is even more beneficial for both psychological and physical health, for people of all ages. There is evidence that giving children more frequent breaks to play outside, such as four 15-minute recesses a day, improves behavior and school performance.[463] Spending time outside also helps children with ADHD, and in particular, park-based programs improve test scores, self-discipline, and behavior.[464] [465] [466] [467]

Adults Can Become Technology-addicted Too

These same principles apply to adults, but we often use our powers of rationalization to minimize perceived benefits, especially when they go against our preconceived notions of success or our lifestyle preferences. As we get older, we may be less likely to seek out time in nature, even if we've had good experiences in the past. Thankfully, more studies on adults are forthcoming, which may create a good basis for physicians to write "forest prescriptions" for adults as well as for children. Even bringing nature into and around our homes and work areas is helpful; small things like making sure to open windows frequently and caring for indoor plants can improve air quality, and spending time growing an outside garden can be wonderfully rewarding and beneficial.

Now even public health and environmental health professionals are collaborating more frequently and coming up with excellent advice for creating natural spaces that improve physical and mental health for humans.[468] [469] One of my favorite forms of meditation, which is becoming increasingly popular, is Japanese "forest bathing," and versions of it are beginning to appear in the U.S.[470] [471] [472] The idea is simple: just spend time quietly listening in the woods, whether this is half an hour outside in a park near your home or getting out of the city for a few hours to a deep forest or other natural area. Health benefits have been found to extend up to a month after the forest trip, and presumably effects will be cumulative and longer lasting the more one spends time in the forest.

Similarly, researchers are finding that resetting the circadian rhythm using natural light is beneficial to health. Exercising in the early morning light improves weight loss, as does keeping a circadian schedule through the weekends instead of significantly changing one's sleep schedule, which causes what has been termed "social jet lag."[473] [474] This means sleeping in on the weekends might be helpful to catch up on sleep, but only if not combined with later than usual bedtimes. Technology can help bring Sustainable Health principles into your life too, as evidenced in studies on computer programs designed to help depressed patients improve sleep hygiene and circadian rhythm, which has helped reduce symptoms significantly.[475]

The scientific community is becoming more interested in finding ways of integrating people and nature back together to improve health, and although many areas require a good deal more study, the general direction is promising.[476] Planning city layouts and public transportation with human relationships and health in mind is not only sustainable, but a way to cause faster economic and positive environmental change, since cities are smaller and more maneuverable politically than states or countries. Studies on transportation alternatives to personal car use (including bikes, city trains, and buses) and traffic patterns (such as roundabouts, protected bike lanes, more bike parking, and dedicated center turn lanes) consistently show that improving the "greenness" of transportation systems also improves the local economy. Starting locally and demonstrating that interventions work for social, economic, and environmental justice helps provide larger institutions like states and countries with proven scalable alternatives.

Changes in work hours for adults are being experimented with, too. Shorter workdays are associated with more productivity, and especially for doctors and nurses, shorter workdays with longer appointment times are catching on, bringing better results for both doctors and patients.[477] [478] [479] Less time spent sitting, as we talked about in chapter 8, is helpful for numerous health reasons. With shorter workdays and more time spent with family and outdoors, making better health choices overall is much more likely when one has time to rest well and exercise.

10

EMBRACING UNCERTAINTY

Telling doctors to embrace uncertainty probably sounds like a type of blasphemy. From the first science class in elementary school, it seems as if there is an answer to anything we could ask, and if not, one will be found if we just look hard enough. This remains true for many of us, even during medical school. When we don't understand something, we go further into the sciences to investigate. We assume there is an answer, even if it might take years to find. By the time we get into residency, we are thoroughly steeped in the paradigm of "I'll find out, sir," and respond the same way every time a patient or attending asks us something we don't know. Even when things go wrong, when patients get sicker with treatment, or die unexpectedly, we assume a mistake was made, that we missed something, or at least next time the answer will be clearer, if we look more closely, are more vigilant. In the real world, not only do we make mistakes that are sometimes deadly, but sometimes clear explanations never come.

Doctors are trained in medical school and in our culture that they are supposed to find THE answer—and to be "right." Doctors' sense of self-worth is often bound tightly to their problem-solving ability, their ability to reach for an answer that will help, and their ability to be right. When something a doctor says is questioned by patients or other practitioners, many doctors I know tend to react with anger (or at least derision) before even considering the question fully. When we doctors are unsure, but still need to make a decision about a diagnosis or treatment plan, our sense of rightness protects our egos and carries us over the hump of indecision. When we're wrong, sometimes it's hard to admit or even look at objectively. Added to this is the pervasive cultural assumption our patients share: there is always a right answer. And so, we have arrived in the current quagmire of malpractice fears and a tail-covering practice of medicine.

This science-based need to be right has grown to leviathan proportions in about the same time frame as our difficulties with discussing and expecting death. Being wrong or not knowing the answer is almost as terrifying as staring death in the face and saying, "Okay, you win." Because of our idea that our job is to fight death and disease, failure to understand what happened can feel as bad as "losing" to death. Joanne Lynn, a researcher of end-of-life issues, says in Atul Gawande's great book *Being Mortal*, "People used to experience life-threatening illness like bad weather… you either got through it or you didn't."[480]

Before antibiotics and our current arsenal of other medications, doctors used to know better when there was nothing they could do, because that happened more often. They were often better able to admit it, let it go, and lay the blame with fate or God. Now that there is nearly always another pill or treatment to try, that feeling of resignation or helplessness usually only arises during an actual "code blue"—when someone has had CPR for a while and the drugs or chest compressions aren't working. If we were to stop offering excessive treatments any earlier, or question whether going on in the expected way will be of benefit, our training leads us to feel we've failed and not tried hard enough. Malpractice insurance is astronomical for the same reason, since patients have bought into this as well and often put the blame of any bad outcome squarely on their doctor's shoulders.

I'm not saying malpractice doesn't happen, of course it does, but the fear of it and the habit of ordering unnecessary tests to make sure the medical record looks like the doctors have "done enough," is not helpful to patients or to our medical system. The reality is that we actually might never know 90 percent of the reasons why someone becomes ill or gets better. Yes, we can of course make extremely well-educated guesses. Yes, we can observe apparent causes in each patient's history and apparent effects from the medicines we give. But we can't know with 100 percent certainty—ever.

The medical literature overflows with evidence of this. Most medicines work moderately well in a third of the people with the illness the drug is meant for, a third of the people experience side effects, and a third experience almost no effect. Some medicines, like pills to increase bone density, are now known to cause rare but much stranger fractures than those they were designed to prevent, because they don't strengthen bone the structural way normal healing does—they mostly make it thicker. "Paradoxical" reactions, where patients have the opposite reaction to the drug than the one expected (think of children who become extra energetic with antihistamines like Benadryl instead of slightly sedated), and severe, adverse reactions (like hallucinations from fluoroquinolone antibiotics) happen relatively often but without apparent or predictable reason.

Unexpected and unpredictable results happen outside of medications as well. MRI scans of spines in people with and without back pain show abnormalities in discs and vertebrae that don't correlate with pain. Guidelines for cancer screenings change almost yearly, because as more statistics become available, the evidence is uncertain as to the benefits of many types of screenings we've depended on for decades; often the screening leads to too many false positives and doesn't catch enough cancers to be valuable for the entire population. Guidelines for medications change frequently too, and different preventative task force organizations can sometimes make opposing recommendations, leaving patients and doctors to decide which of the recommendations are most worth following.[481] [482]

Recommendations for managing chronic diseases change frequently, too. For instance, current blood pressure recommendations come from the "JNC 8" report, which is the eighth official recommendation of the Joint National Committee and based on findings about preventing blood-pressure-related illnesses like heart attacks and strokes. The JNC comes out when experts perceive new guidelines are necessary; the last one, "JNC 7," was published in 2003. This means that as medicines and epidemiology have improved, recommendations have changed eight times since 1976 when the first report came out. Suggestions for supplements change even faster, and while most show no evidence of benefit over time, many are found to be harmful years later. Dr. Vinayak Prasad and Dr. Adam Cifu recently wrote a great book about this concept, *Ending Medical Reversal: Improving Outcomes, Saving Lives*, calling for the requirement of better evidence before medications are approved and guidelines made official.[483]

The reason for all of this uncertainty seems obvious to me, after years of both "success" and "failure" in my practice of medicine. The systems of the human body are as complex as the planet's ecosystems. While our science is much better now than it was even 20 years ago, it seems the more mysteries we uncover and the more details we discover, the more questions spring up in their places. Because there are still so many unanswered questions, and because we don't yet know the significance or true utility of many recent discoveries, it is important to be critical and careful with the science we use. It is vital to check in with scholars in the humanities and with our own moral compasses to make sure we aren't only doing what's most expedient in the moment, but also that we're taking care of both people and the planet in ways that will not harm future generations.

Seeing People as "Happenings"—Slow Medicine

Because we can't know everything, and because more often than we'd like patients don't respond or present in ways that make immediate sense, and/or the medical system doesn't have the answers we want or need, it helps to pause when things aren't as simple as we thought. In addition to using science carefully, it is useful to step back regularly, let go of the need to be right for a moment, and see patients as a miraculous "happening," as Alan Watts would say; a happening that includes all their ancestors, how they were brought up, the food they've eaten and eat now, athletic choices, how "dirty" their childhoods might or might not have been, what sleep pattern is typical, what they do for a living now or earlier, what their philosophy of life is, how polluted is the air and water nearby, and do they feel fulfilled? There is actually never a true discrete cause or effect for anything at all. Every event we think we see is preceded by every variable that led to it, and every event we think we see is followed by an infinite number of effects we will never know about. Stepping back and taking the time to see a patient as this type of dance with past and future is what Dr. Victoria Sweet calls "slow medicine" in her book *God's Hotel*.[484] Despite taking more time, this approach ends up, in her view and mine, being a more efficient way of practicing medicine.

Today, doctors are required to quickly skim a chart and then are only able to deal with one symptom or issue during a seven-minute visit. If instead, doctors have time to find out more about an individual patient's variables, with time to let those variables marinate with all the knowledge we've gained in school and in practice, it is much more likely that solutions will be found. If there is time to dialogue with the patient, it is more likely that treatment plans will be agreed upon together and that they will be much more effective. And, as will be discussed in the next chapter, if doctors and patients know each other well, it is more likely that both will be better able to come to terms with the unknown. Especially when medical solutions are unavailable, both sides understand that "everything has been done," and the conversation can focus on prioritizing and making the most of the time that is left.

In the long run, slow medicine means more illnesses can be prevented, more chronic diseases can be reversed, and countless dollars in health care costs can be saved—along with lives. Much of this can be done with attention to each patient's lifestyle and diet, removing things that are harmful (poor sleep, diet, stressful behavior patterns) and adding things that are helpful (exercise, stress management, whole food nutrition, and medications only when necessary). Slow medicine is more sustainable medicine. This is the principle ecologists use in many ecosystems in peril from human intervention: remove the destructive process if possible and allow nature to heal itself with reasonable interventional help. The reason this works is that there is rarely a single cause, and never only one effect, of an illness or treatment. But going back to basics like sleep, food, and movement encourages the body's self-healing mechanisms to work as efficiently as possible, doing the type of work that many of our medications attempt to mimic.

I find it particularly strange that doctors are taught in medical school that "lifestyle and diet" advice is always the first-line treatment for "lifestyle diseases," and in theory, medicines are only to be used when that has "failed," yet in practice, lifestyle advice is mentioned with a flippant attitude that suggests "no one can do those things." The truth is, medical school classes emphasize medicines, standardized diet recommendations, and how tightly the guidelines say to try to control out-of-whack lab values. Med students are told how many different medications can be piled on "safely," and which medications will counter side effects of other medications. Most of us eventually realize that although blood pressure medicines reduce high blood pressure, they don't remove it, and although insulin saves lives, it doesn't fix insulin resistance permanently. We might instead start to teach individualized treatment plans that could allow us to "fix" these types of problems more permanently, or at least slow them down.

There's a trend in both Western and "alternative" medicine circles these days that revolves around practitioners, authors, and "health gurus" using the phrase "root cause of illness." I have done that in the past, too, so I understand the idea behind this current fad. It starts with the premise that the current medical system is a symptom-management and emergency medicine machine, which is not untrue. It is true that there are causes for high blood pressure, insomnia, diabetes, obesity, and psychological problems beyond what the usual dogma suggests and far beyond what government and insurance companies measure for "quality assurance" in health care. It is also true that pills rarely reverse or fix underlying causes of symptoms that may be life threatening, with the exception of some infections and gene therapies. Medicines often function as only a band-aid or stopgap measure for chronic problems like high blood pressure, high blood sugar, heart failure, or poor kidney function. Some of the "root causes" listed by health gurus and marketed in books and membership programs definitely reach deeper than surface symptoms, since changing habits of exercise, diet, sleep, and improving the microbiome all have undeniable health benefits, even in seriously ill people.

However, this is where the root cause fallacy comes in. New discoveries about epigenetics, the microbiome, and neurochemicals happen almost daily, and it's incredibly tempting with each new study about X to say, "This is why Y happens! We just need to study how to make a pill to alter this part of the microbiome/ genome/brain chemistry!" New studies on diet and fasting and metabolism appear frequently as well, and it's tempting to say things such as, "Fasting extends life! Just eat an extremely low-calorie diet and all your health problems will disappear!" (For more information about healthy ways to practice fasting, see appendix 3, and to read more on diet fads, see appendix 2.) New studies on medication side effects, plastic chemical leaching, and pollution emerge regularly as well, and shortly afterwards, someone will always be heard yelling from rooftops, "Chemicals are bad! Use only natural remedies!"

These types of fallacies are just as ridiculous as assuming that because one medicine works for one person, it will fix a similar symptom for another. But since physicians are trained to solve complex problems and find answers, when something is found that looks like a cause that could be changed, we get our claws in and have a very hard time letting go. This is one of the reasons so many doctors and other health-interested people market so many diets, exercise plans, and life-altering programs, and also why people spend so much money on them.

As we've talked about in every chapter, the human body is so complex that it's absurd to imagine we can ever know all the variables responsible for every symptom or illness that arises. Everything can be described as a "chemical," so "natural" doesn't necessarily mean healthy or helpful. Nearly everything can be a medicine or a poison depending on the amount, even oxygen and water. The number of variables affecting health increases exponentially the wider your lens. Assuming we "know" anything from one study, or even several studies, and assuming we should do for everyone what each of those studies conclude is presumptuous and poor science. Since few studies include different races, genders, or people who are pregnant, very old, or very young, many findings aren't likely applicable to the general population anyway. In the end, the reality is that we may never find out what causes some things. Every health guru who says they know the root cause of everyone's issues and will sell you the answer frustrates me to no end.

Yes, some people will benefit from their advice, maybe upwards of 30 percent, similar to the benefits from many medicines, and similar to the placebo effect. And some of these scientists studying newer fields like epigenetics may find out exceptionally helpful information. But microbiome dysfunction can be hereditary[485] as well as having epigenetic consequences in the present, affected by diet, exercise, pollution in the environment, and even mood. A new 2017 study suggests that high salt intake (as happens with processed foods) decreases certain gut bacteria and raises blood pressure.[486] Obesity is so multifactorial, with pieces of the puzzle including antibiotics, the microbiome, plastics, pesticides, pollution, food, exercise, sleep, trauma, medications, and hormone and neurochemical alterations, that finding one root cause is not possible. Osteoarthritis has multiple and often unrecognized influences, including longstanding minor postural abnormalities, physical trauma, weight, inflammation, food, exercise, genetics, as well as microbiome and hormonal contributions.

In short, everyone who says there is a single root cause of someone's main medical issue, and that their answer is THE answer, keeps us in the "there's a pill for that" mindset, and can pull us away from the more complete healing that might be more likely if we took a wider view.

A Need to Look Deeper

Looking for a root cause can be a good exercise, much like taking a pill to buy time for a chronic illness. It buys time to make lifestyle changes that might make the medication unnecessary later. However, we have to acknowledge that we may never know exactly what caused a symptom or illness. Nor will we ever know the full effects of choices we make, whether we've turned off helpful or harmful genes, and what we may have triggered or avoided by chance or by choice. Stepping back and looking deeper *will* get us farther down a path of healing, by helping illuminate those behaviors and choices that are most helpful—and most harmful. Then we can begin to swing our choices to the more helpful behaviors.

Prioritizing by medical issue will be your best guide regarding where to start. This means focusing on sugar elimination, if pre-diabetes or obesity is your primary and most pressing difficulty, and optimizing sleep and stress management first, if a more serious illness has developed—all while taking the medication prescribed to buy time and control symptoms.

What is less helpful is listening primarily to magic bullet hawkers that claim to know the root cause of your illness and have the tools to treat you. Not that they can't be of help; clearly many of these programs have a good percentage of beneficial information and teach effective ways of allowing the body to start healing itself. But most plans out there aren't well supported by evidence, even if sold by a "doctor" of any stripe. Anything that requires numerous supplements or high fees for access to "healing secrets" is unlikely to be more than a moneymaker for the person selling the programs. No matter how convincing someone is, absolutely no one has all the answers or can cure anything "in 30 days" or "easily" or "without changing your diet" or "with this one weird trick," as so many internet ads say, enticing you to click on them.

Medical practitioners should be ashamed of themselves for using their authority and reputation to tout remedies by using bad science. If one believes something works, that's completely up to each person, but calling oneself a medical practitioner of any kind and then using one's professional authority and questionable science to back up one's stance degrades science in the eyes of the public, and makes it less likely that good science and good doctors will be believed or noticed when their recommendations might save lives or change the course of global health for the better.

I won't go far into the placebo effect here (which is effective over 60 percent of the time, depending on the situation) or spontaneous healing (which does occur, and we have no concrete explanation why most of the time), because those solutions just don't work for everyone. But if your personal path is to find a faith healer or take a "miracle plant" for your cancer and it works,

I will be the first to admit I have no idea why it worked, and the first to celebrate with you the fact that it did. More frequently though, and as I'll go into more in the next chapter, hope based on incorrect information can prevent people from helping themselves with available treatments that might be more effective for them or might align better with their true priorities for their quality of life.

Supplements and Snake Oil

I am obviously exceptionally conservative with recommendations when it comes to pseudoscience or partial science being used to promote products or health programs. One of the best examples of this is the supplement conversation. I can't tell you how many patients I've helped save money on supplements that aren't proven, or at least weren't proven for the reasons they were taking the products. The biggest problem I see is that many of the companies marketing these products use partially accurate science to back up health claims. They simply leap from studies' partially researched hypotheses all the way to dramatic conclusions.

Recently the Academy of Integrative Health and Medicine supported in their newsletter a nutrition expert who gave a talk aimed at doctors about supplements. He cited mountains of data and was meticulous in his presentation. He was absolutely sure that most Americans have low levels of measurable nutrients in their blood, that most are undernourished, and that this can and should be fixed by taking supplements to raise those blood levels. To his credit he did mention that not all brands are created equally, and he did disclose that he works for four supplement companies. I do not argue with the fact that many Americans are undernourished and over-fed. I do not argue that low levels of nutrients might indicate poor health, or that higher levels might be indicative of better health. I could pick apart the amounts of nutrients given and how much they actually raised blood levels, since for many it wasn't appreciable, but the main thing I took issue with was his leap of logic from hypothesis to conclusion using his data.

The problem with his extensive use of data to prove his point was that none of it actually proves that a higher blood level of any vitamin achieved by a supplement improves quality or length of life or stops symptoms of any illness. Not one study cited even looked at that outcome. But improving quality or length of life is generally what people who take vitamins and supplements are after. This is a huge disconnect! Most studies that do look at health outcomes related to vitamins or supplements find that when people eat the **food** associated with those vitamins, they are indeed protected from some diseases and do live longer and healthier lives. Particularly in the cases of antioxidants, vitamin D, vitamin E, calcium, and omega-3 fatty acids, the data points to food sources as protective, whereas supplements are equivocal at best, harmful at worst. For example, vitamin C hasn't been proven to cure anything except actual scurvy. We know diets high in vitamin C are helpful, but those diets are high in other vitamins as well. For instance, in apples, vitamin C accounts for only 0.4 percent of the total (excellent) antioxidant activity of the whole fruit.[487]

In some cases, especially when specific supplements can't be obtained from food, taking a particular compound separately *can* be helpful. But even in these cases, often a smaller amount of a supplement works better for relief of symptoms than a higher dose, as with oil supplements for knee arthritis.[488] In other cases, adding a vitamin to a food which lacks it naturally seems a good idea but totally fails to live up to expectations, like in the case of vitamin A being genetically added to rice, which failed to live up to expected improvements in rates of blindness in children. Instead, other factors such as improved breastfeeding rates and food diversification led to the documented improvements all over Southeast Asia over a more than 20-year period.[489] [490]

Good quality of life outcomes are proven for only a tiny fraction of supplements, and higher blood levels don't necessarily relate to tissue absorption or use. These outcomes and the reasons for this are particularly difficult to assess in people with genetic deletions and other genetic variants related to vitamin uptake, as well as those with digestive difficulties. For instance, there is a fairly common mutation in the MTHFR gene, which can decrease the ability to use regular folate (vitamin B9) found in plants like leafy greens. Taking too much supplemental folate, or synthetic folic acid if you cannot process folate, is extra concerning, however, since supplementation of folic acid has been associated with certain cancers like prostate and lung. Keep in mind that FOOD intake of folic acid is associated with *decreased* cancer risk, and supplementation is still necessary during pregnancy.

Since too much of a good thing really can be harmful, particularly with fat-soluble vitamins, supplements might be more dangerous than we would think regarding something marketed as "healthy." What we do know about supplements so far is discouraging, and the available evidence doesn't point toward recommending them to everyone. Especially in patients with multiple health conditions or on medications, it is concerning that use of supplements has increased without much data showing benefit, and very little showing side effects or harms.[491]

The bottom line for this particular topic has two parts that are mirrored in many other subtopics in medicine. First, we're not sure how to accurately measure *functional* levels of many of the vitamins and minerals in people's bodies. Second, we're not sure of the best way to correct all nutritional deficiencies, much less the symptoms of health problems that we aren't sure are *causally* associated with these deficiencies in the first place. (This obviously does not include deficiencies that are well known and were historically the reason we discovered the existence of several vitamins, like C for scurvy, D for rickets, B3 for pellagra, B1 for beri beri, etc.)

Until we have good outcome measures on all the marketed products out there, improved nutrition from whole foods is the safest way to improve nutritional status.[492] [493] Taking the chemical components out of food and ingesting them in large doses will likely have different and at times very negative effects, especially since we don't yet know all of the components of every food that are beneficial or negative, or how to combine them to best effect. This includes all the heavily marketed vitamins, freeze-dried pills of fruits and vegetables, and "green drinks," as none of these are proven to increase longevity, protect from cancer, or benefit health in general. So, it is best to simply eat the whole food rather than a chemically isolated component of the food. Pseudo-science and incomplete science should not be used to assume cause or effect relating to human health, and certainly should not be used to promote any product or health program. Health does not need to cost as much as the hundred billion dollar supplement industry would have you believe.

It is, of course, hard to police pseudoscience, and the huge amount of it available on the internet makes most physicians loathe to even *consider* information patients find online or through marketing of books and programs. But because of the prevailing cultural belief around health, I've heard both patients and doctors exclaim in frustration: "There must be something you can prescribe to fix this!" And when doctors don't know or aren't sure what would help, people tend to turn to another "expert," which nowadays usually means Someone On The Internet. In these cases, both doctors and patients need to keep in mind our overall lack of understanding of how the human body really heals itself and what risks and benefits might affect a given patient at a given time. Every week there are hidden health risks uncovered and previous health risks declared healthy, from the water poisoning crisis in Flint, Michigan, and the DuPont chemical cover-up in Parkersburg, West Virginia,[494] to news about cheese improving nutrition[495] [496] and high dose vitamin D possibly worsening falls in the elderly.[497] Starting out with whole foods, optimized sleep, and regular exercise will likely get us farther than any expensive plan we can find online.

Uncertainty is Best Faced With an Integrative Approach

When one wants to do everything possible to become or stay healthy, to prevent or reverse disease, or to fight a devastating diagnosis, it is frustrating to try to sift through available information, especially when Western medicine has fallen short. But before throwing the baby out with the bath water, both doctors and patients need to step back and really look at the uncertainty of the situation at hand. It isn't necessary to give up on science, nor to disregard alternative theories of health improvement.

Lately I've seen many heartening examples of traditional science (at least science in the last 100 years) and more holistic thinking working together to exponentially help patients. In programs and policies for dealing with drug addicts, decriminalization is both more economical and leads to more successful rehabilitation in some cases.[498] Instead of further marginalizing the homeless and treating many with drug problems or mental illness in emergency rooms or prisons, simply giving them housing and better access to services saves cities and states huge amounts of money, which is not only a more compassionate approach but also a more financially responsible one.[499] [500] [501] Instead of prescribing or marketing diets with the certainty that each practitioner's opinion is "The Answer" to cancer, diabetes, heart disease, or anything else, individual genetic and microbial differences mean individualized diets will likely be more helpful in the future. Good research is even being done on the placebo effect, even though it is incredibly hard to study accurately, and doctors are catching on and wanting to harness patients' mind-body healing power.[502]

There are examples of unexpected discoveries changing rapidly how we understand and hopefully how we will treat some illnesses that have continued to baffle us, like the role of synaptic pruning going awry in schizophrenia.[503] Then there are alarming examples of how, by changing something we think is harmful, we may end up worse off than with the original problem, as in the case of BPA and BPA alternatives being used in food packaging (plastics and tin can linings). It turns out the new alternatives may not be an improvement at all.[504] If we expect miracles along with disappointments, taking a more pragmatic and rather Zen approach to medicine, our collective levels of frustration decrease—as well as our tendency to grasp at straws.

Embracing uncertainty helps both patients and doctors, and it allows us to get away from the "there's a pill for that" mentality, while keeping us from despairing when many of the usual treatments are ineffective. Knowing there might not be an answer makes it possible to let go of needing to be right, to consider options that might not be obvious, and to take time to allow creative solutions to come forward. Educated guesses are reasonable, and practicing medicine involves science as well as subjectivity, but doctors need to use guidelines from good science as *guides* rather than laws, since each patient is different and has different priorities. Becoming better friends with the fact that none of us are in control and can't know the answers to everything can help doctors just as much as patients, as the number of doctors and medical students with depression and suicidal thoughts and behaviors continues to rise.[505] Doctors are more likely to be burned out and unhappy and more likely to change professions than any other vocation.[506] Understanding the fact that there might not be an answer, finding peace with that within oneself, then using that knowledge to take the time to get to know each other better, regardless of outcome, is more valuable perhaps than all the science and schooling available.

11

DEATH

Just as I started making arrangements to have space to start writing this book, Atul Gawande's book *Being Mortal: Medicine and What Matters in the End* arrived in my reading list.[507] The book resonated with me for two reasons. First, in my Internal Medicine residency, I occasionally was called "the hospice queen." The term got thrown around mostly during ICU or geriatrics rotations—where hospice was more often part of our care options, given that we saw proportionally more people die then—so hospice and death were on my mind a lot. Second, I had personally gone through two difficult deaths.

My grandfather, like his mother before him, spent the last few of his 92 years wishing "God would take him." Due to severe anxiety, depression, deafness, cataracts, and arthritis, his sense of despair eventually overrode his naturally gregarious and adventurous personality. These blocks to communication with others accelerated his dementia, making his last year full of frustration and conflict. That the conflicts might have been avoided, or at least lessened, never entered the minds of his primary caregivers, despite my mother's and my attempts at trying to head off those issues before they became severe. And had his doctors had more experience with geriatric medicine and end-of-life considerations, preparations for more comfortable care could have been started long before that last difficult year, when logical conversations with him were no longer possible.

Much of Dr. Gawande's book was not news to me, but I learned about some great projects in terminal and elderly care that I wished I had known about during residency. *Being Mortal* is so well done that I hope it is now required reading not only in medical schools but also for students of nursing, physician assistants, and other professional health care providers. There are some great statistics there as well, so I won't go into too much depth here research-wise. I would like to explain, particularly to medical students, before most of them have had to deal head-on with patients dying in front of them, why it is of the utmost importance to think about death frequently, clearly, and with a sense of gratitude. Becoming friends with death will make your practice of medicine better, and will also help develop a deeper sense of peace personally.

When my mother died during my intern year, from both cancer and mismanagement of her case, it took a while for the early shock to wear off. But when it did, and I'd worked through the worst of the early grief, I found I was much more attuned to patients' experiences of death. These two very different, very personal, examples of how death can happen pushed me to really pay attention to how the medical system deals with death—and even more, how it doesn't.

It may seem nonsensical to point this out, but if natural death never occurred, life would be horrific. Life could not even exist without death—we would quickly run out of resources. When some things pass away, new things are allowed to begin. This is true in a physical sense and also in a philosophical sense. We are part of the natural world, and in nature, death allows growth, learning, and evolution, even if it's not on a timeline we can easily perceive. For humans especially, death can bring a sense of immediacy and gratitude for the time we have.

This may be less obvious, but simply living longer isn't necessarily desirable. If you ask a sick patient with three months to live if they want another month, many of them will hesitate and ask how much obtaining that extra month would cost. If chemotherapy would make every day full of doctors, nausea, and pain, then some people might choose to live the three months they were given as an estimate without chemotherapy—just with good pain control and possibly more family time. It depends on all sorts of things, but these considerations are absolutely necessary to think through. Living *longer* is rarely the actual goal, if our desires are carefully examined, but living *better* generally is.

This is something I didn't understand before my mother became ill. I remember her asking me (three weeks before she died, over the phone while I was on call, 800 miles away), "What should I do?" Her choices, as it appeared to me at the time, were either to "try" or to "give up." I remember how angry I was with her for even considering "giving up." In the codependence of a single-mother/only-child situation, I didn't want her to "decide" to leave me, from a subconscious point of view. As if it were her choice. In retrospect, it was unfair of her to depend on me for that decision, and it was ridiculous of me to think I had a good answer for her. But this subconscious reaction to death and illness is the most common way we, as people steeped in Western culture, make decisions.

Because my mother's medical team at a famous teaching/research hospital had changed over the week before, they didn't know her. They couldn't answer her questions, didn't deal well with her side effects or pain, and almost daily confused her with her neighbor in the room next door who had the same first name. Not that I blame her team directly of course—her new resident was only a year ahead of me in training and was considerably less interested in patient care than I was, favoring book learning and presumably applying for research fellowships.

Meanwhile, my mom's attending doctor had a huge number of patients to oversee, and my mother's case didn't fit into a normal diagnosis/treatment paradigm. The medical response to her condition was to give her chemotherapy for both types of cancers they believed she had, and to see if they could get her prepared for a bone marrow transplant, which they thought would likely cure her.

Knowing what I know now, I can see what happened more clearly. My mother was not a physically strong person. She was overweight, undernourished, chronically depressed for years, and wickedly intelligent, but disconnected from and disappointed in her physical body. She valued time with family, independence, and her religion. She hated MRI machines and medicines and didn't care for most healthy food. She had survived brain tumor surgery at 30, a double mastectomy for breast cancer at 45, and had been living in severe pain with undertreated rheumatoid arthritis for five years prior to her cancer diagnosis.

To me, this gave her the equivalent of at least three "co-morbidities" (pre-existing and complicating health problems) at the time of her diagnosis. In the care of older patients, the more medical problems a patient has, the less well they are likely to do in surgery. If an emergency happens in the hospital and CPR is performed on someone with more than one medical problem, the likelihood they will walk out of the hospital is near zero. The same applies to chemotherapy, which is an incredibly traumatic assault on the entire body, one that even strong, young patients sometimes do not survive.

My mom had already quit her volunteer job teaching Sunday school at her church, and when her bone marrow dysfunction became critical and a bone marrow transplant was suggested, she quit her high-powered job and moved to be closer to her father, brother, and his family. The first night she was to spend in her new apartment, a painful fever overtook her in the afternoon, and she was taken to the hospital. It was discovered that the leukemia they had diagnosed her with via bone marrow testing was now accompanied by a seemingly separate lymphoma, which was acute and required immediate chemotherapy. The doctors still believed a bone marrow transplant would fix both problems, but they needed to give her chemotherapy for both types of cancer at the same time.

Her first resident was amazing, a third year who was hoping to be an oncologist himself. While I visited during her first week, after I'd seen him a few days in a row, I took him aside. I asked if I should quit my residency and stay with her. I asked him if her condition looked "bad" to him, if he thought she would survive this. He paused and really thought about his answer. He took a deep breath and calmly told me when his father had terminal cancer, he quit everything and spent time with him, and it was the best decision he had made. He said he couldn't predict what might happen, but that was his experience, and he hoped my mom would do well.

Despite his excellent advice, my brain latched onto the hope part of his comment. He warned me about the different personalities of next week's physician team, and that I'd need to be vigilant about getting information, and he said he wished he could stay on the team for my mom. He was the kindest, smartest, and most compassionate physician I have ever encountered in relation to my family. I am so grateful I have that bright spot to look back on, even if I didn't take the best part of his advice. In the aftermath, his was the voice I remember, and it was he whom I decided I wanted to emulate as I continued my residency.

The next three weeks were pretty terrible. My mother stopped being able to eat, and had severe diarrhea and abdominal pain. Her chemotherapy agents were not discontinued or paused. Along with the severe pain, one day she developed a dangerous heart rhythm, and was transferred to the ICU. After a few days her rhythm stabilized, but her doctors had trouble explaining what the next course of action would be over the phone to me while I was on a busy ICU rotation myself, 800 miles to the south.

Her pain continued, and her emotions started veering wildly away from her usual intellectual melancholy, peppered by occasional anger and general good humor. She would cry on the phone to me, and I would then try to get her attending physician to call me back. She was miserable, and I had no idea what to do. Being an intern, I simply didn't have the experience to understand what was happening, and being her daughter, what was clearly going on a few states away was too hard for my heart to handle, so I stayed firmly in a state of denial disguised as hope.

On her last night, before my emergency flight home, she had a seizure, and during my conversation with her brother who had called to tell me, he said she was trying to take off her heart monitor. Having seen patients do this in the hours before they died, I automatically sprang into what I call my "ICU mode." I held firmly to my medical knowledge, got a hold of the doctor on call, and tried to find out what had happened. The extremely perceptive and excellent on-call resident agreed to order blood tests that hadn't been done in a week, and to discontinue the new medication that had been started that day, an antidepressant that helps with chronic pain, presumably because she was still crying in pain constantly. But as I found out the next morning, she was also delirious with undiagnosed liver failure and in pain due to typhlitis, which is intestinal inflammation associated with low white blood cell counts. I suspect that was the undiagnosed cause of her pain that had started three weeks prior, while I was still visiting. She also had intestinal bleeding, but because they didn't know her at all, despite seeing her daily for three weeks, the doctors had decided the cause of her abdominal pain and confusion was depression.

The on-call doctor the night before I flew in was amazing, competent, and just as frustrated as I was with the situation. But at that point neither of us had any power to change the outcome. The next morning, I rushed from the airport to the hospital and arrived to find my mother with yellow skin, in agonal breathing, about to be intubated, and completely unconscious. She was on "contact precautions" from one of her infections, so I wasn't allowed to touch her.

I remember standing by her bed, saying words I don't remember now, knowing she couldn't hear me, and then walking out of the room in shock to allow the doctors to put the tube into her lungs. Somehow, after pressing her resident to show me her lab results from the night before, after going over her values and tests not ordered during the previous week, and accepting that they completely missed her liver failure, I for some reason agreed when they said her altered mental status was from cancer in her brain fluid, and okayed a spinal injection of chemotherapy. She died less than an hour after that injection while in the MRI machine.

Learning from Death—or—Allowing Myself to Be Taught

To say I wasn't prepared for my mother's death would be the biggest understatement of all time. Fortunately, my mother's brother was her executor, and I had work to return to, so I sublimated my absolute inability to cope into furious learning. When the dust started to clear, and after two close friends helped me through the worst of it, I threw myself into knowledge acquisition and a desire to become the best doctor possible. I wanted to know everything—to do as much as I could to prevent pain, disease, and death. Well, maybe not death…

It took time, patients' deaths, and arguments with my attendings, but I gradually understood that what had happened with my mother was not a necessary outcome. The final outcome— her dying much earlier than expected—would have happened without any medical intervention, but the suffering leading up to it could have been alleviated or avoided entirely. Learning about hospice from amazing social workers and other physicians, I started to imagine a wider range of possibilities aside from 1) fighting or 2) giving up. I could see that instead of four weeks of chemotherapy and misery in the hospital, she may have been more content and at peace if I had suggested taking her to Hawaii, her favorite beautiful place, and being around horses, a dream she'd had since childhood. If that adventure wasn't possible, maybe time with her family and comfort food would have sufficed. Maybe or maybe not, but without having that discussion, her priorities and mine were never shared, so simple pain and grief from illness and death became suffering instead.

Accepting this was what taught me to look deeper when treating my patients. I realized I had to get to know them better, to know their families, their religion, their understanding of death. And even if the patients themselves were delirious or unconscious, my job was the same: to seriously evaluate what possible outcomes were available and likely, to be clear and honest with the family, and to try to do the least harm if the patient was to have a chance to walk out of the hospital back to the functional life they had before.

I remember a patient I'll call Mr. Flores. He was a handsome and incredibly tall man. A neighbor had found him in his apartment, surrounded by alcohol bottles and his own waste. The term "skin and bones" never applied to anyone more than him, all the more alarming because of his obvious height, despite his inability to sit up. In the ER on CT scan, he was found to have widespread metastatic cancer, likely from his prostate, which had never been treated that we knew of. He was combative, occasionally moaning in pain, but too confused to answer any questions or even give his name. Our medical team and social worker tried to find his family, but no one called us back. It was clear to me that his time was short, and that given the way he was found, he might have been ready to die and certainly wanted to be free of pain.

I asked my attending physician two days in a row to help me sign his chart with a "double doc," which is a colloquial term we use when two doctors sign together to make a decision for patients who cannot decide for themselves. Having two doctors sign means, in theory, that the medical team has asked for outside opinion and done as much as possible to make the best medical decision for the patient's benefit. I wished to make him medically a Do Not Resuscitate (DNR) patient, since nothing we could do aside from comfort care would help him at his late stage of disease, and it would be criminal and futile to perform CPR, breaking his ribs and hurting him to try to resuscitate him should his heart or breathing stop.

The answer I was given was that we should wait longer, and "do everything" until his family was contacted so we could be sure they were okay with that decision. I replied that the decision was soon not going to be ours to make, that he had very little time left. Mr. Flores' nurses had a very hard time even administering pain medication, much less the IV fluids and medicines ordered to hopefully help with his confusion. I thought the only reasonable job we could actually accomplish would be to make his last day or so comfortable, clean, and as pain-free as possible.

On his third day, I arrived at the hospital in the early morning, and after getting my list of new patients, I started off to the medical floors for my morning rounds. A friend who was on ICU call the night before met me in the hallway and said he was sorry about my patient. I had no idea which one he meant, and I combed through the list in my head to see who was most likely to have had an emergency the night before. He shocked me by saying Mr. Flores' name. My breath left me as he told me Mr. Flores had started having severe intestinal bleeding, his blood pressure had dropped, and his heart stopped. He had been taken to the ICU, per hospital protocol for patients not designated as DNR or "comfort care," and after several rounds of CPR and 10 pints of blood, he was declared dead.

I was so upset I couldn't speak to my attending that day beyond yes or no answers. I had trouble with the anger I felt when

I imagined Mr. Flores being put through medical torture in his final hours, hoping he had been unconscious and not in pain during any of it. It was appalling that all that medical expertise, doctors' and nurses' time, and donated blood were spent in futile battle with a death the patient had seemed to want to be quiet and pain-free.

Since my mother's death was still fresh in my mind, I knew I was more upset about this patient's treatment than maybe was reasonable. I can't ever know if I was right about my assumption of how he felt, or if the family might have sued the hospital if we had allowed him to die peacefully. It still seems senseless to me that a medical team isn't allowed to say, "Doing more would only bring pain, doing less is better medicine," and be believed rather than sued.

This incident taught me clearly that today's medical system is not yet set up for realistic and practical—not to mention compassionate—ways of dealing with death and dying. I was a patient advocate before, not hesitating to go as high as necessary to get procedures done for patients who needed them. I was comfortable spending hours in family meetings to make sure everyone was clear on treatment plans, and would take extra time when discharging patients to do my best to prevent misunderstandings about medications and follow-up appointments. But it was Mr. Flores, along with my mother, who made it clear to me why teaching doctors about death and speaking to families about death long before it's imminent is so important.

Improving Quality of Life all the Way to Death

I am not alone in my experiences with the medical system, as a family member or as a physician. Bioethicist Daniel Callahan wrote an excellent commentary and interview with Lisa Krieger, who'd written a moving piece about her father's death and the financial and emotional costs that went with it.[508] They and others have come to some of the same conclusions I have: that quality of life should be the focus, and improved communication is key. Several essays have been written in the last few years about how doctors are emphatic about wanting to die differently than their patients do.[509]

To avoid such awful endings, medical staff and families need to understand that it is sometimes okay to say, "There is nothing more we can do," and that "doing more" is sometimes harmful. Doctors have more experience with death and dying than any other profession, seeing it coming long before it happens. And in the case of primary care doctors outside the hospital, we continue to deal with the aftermath with families for years afterwards. Primary care doctors and specialists alike need to talk with patients about their preferences long before they end up in a hospital, and to do that they need better training in medical school and residency. While some programs are doing well, many still fail miserably to help students understand how to provide truly compassionate care at the end of life.[510]

Ultimately, our whole culture needs a serious overhaul regarding death. As people live longer and the proportion of elderly people continues to increase, we need to address and change the economic impacts of our strange cultural denial of death. The extreme medical costs associated with futile treatment in the last two weeks of life put a huge and unnecessary burden on caregivers and the medical system itself. As medicine gets better at managing illness and saving lives earlier on, and with better management available for chronically and seriously ill patients, those needing more care than their families can supply will need more help maintaining quality of life as their abilities change over time—not just "health and safety" precautions.

This brings me back to Atul Gawande's book. He contends rightly that assisted living and nursing facilities should provide actual "assistance with living," that the avoidance of death is disrespectful of life, and that sometimes the ability to make "poor" or unsafe decisions is not what gives someone a reason to live. One of the most important jobs for doctors should be to find out what is most important to our terminal and elderly patients and facilitate what we can. We should not simply assume that more time is what is desired, but rather we need to look at what our patients consider to be worthwhile. Life extension should not be the ultimate goal, but rather quality and purpose of life. If we go into a conversation about this afraid of death ourselves, or afraid of the patient's or family's reaction to what we will say, we will end up discussing a fantasy based on everyone's "hope" that there won't be an end.

However, I disagree with Dr. Gawande's definition of medicine as "fighting death and disease," because to me, the practice of medicine is assisting with healing, which can happen despite and many times *because of* death and disease. People who are dying, who have the time to come to terms with that fact, are a great gift and have been given a great gift. As Dr. Gawande says, the "role of a dying person" is indeed one of the least appreciated ones in our current culture.

The time to consider death is long before death is imminent, and we shortchange ourselves tremendously as a society by promoting youth and health as the only parts of life to value. We think of success in terms of accumulated wealth or career advancement, but very few people in their last weeks and months wish to receive anything other than love and compassion. As Dr. Gawande mentions, people who are told they have only a short time left often change their priorities. Important issues shift to repairing relationships, passing on their wisdom, spending time with loved ones, and perhaps finishing something or experiencing something that had been put off until time became short.

Many books, articles, and studies have been written in the last few years that have become popular discussion prompters for patients and doctors alike. A very young neurosurgeon who was diagnosed with terminal lung cancer wrote an amazing memoir about his experience with dying, and his wife's subsequent thoughts after his passing are touching and beautiful, instead of only tragic.[511] Most recently, an excellent *The Economist* article about how we think about and deal with death ended with the perfect statement: "Honest and open conversations with the dying should be as much a part of modern medicine as prescribing drugs or fixing broken bones. A better death means a better life, right until the end."[512]

The time for ensuring a peaceful and comfortable exit from this life starts long before a diagnosis of cancer or dementia or the end stage of a chronic disease. But if one is given a diagnosis, there is usually a bit of time to come to terms with it and decide the best course of action. When the first choice of action or treatment might fail, there is often still some time to discuss death as not just a possibility but an expected outcome, even if the next treatment does work well. And as uncomfortable as that conversation can feel, your doctor can be the best person with whom to have that discussion. They've seen more death, helped people die comfortably, fought against the inevitable, and witnessed death by medical treatment more than any other profession. And, if they've been able to learn about death itself from these experiences, rather than count them as wins or losses, they can be more qualified to have these discussions with their patients than most others would be. Discussions about death are not an admission of defeat or denial of hope; honest discussions allow space for more life and more quality choices.

While writing this book, the 96-year-old husband of a patient and friend of mine became seriously ill. I was only able to visit once a week or so, and since her husband was never my patient, I had precious little sway when speaking with his health care team. He did not understand what hospice was, and he had always refused to even discuss it as possibly useful to him. In his delirium, he could not take in new information, but he was occasionally partially lucid, so his health care team would not take his wife's word that his true wishes were to be comfortable and never to be in a hospital or nursing home again. When he came down with pneumonia at home, a home health nurse called an ambulance after less than a minute of being in the house, without speaking to his wife. He spent his last three weeks in the hospital and a nursing home, with excellent care, but he was confused most of the time, agitated, uncomfortable, and constantly begging her to take him home.

The week before he died, although often delirious, he was adamant for a few hours that he needed to speak with his publisher about his children's book, and that he wanted to finish it soon. His few moments of lucidity were filled with love and art, like his previous 96 years, but also frustration that his art was not nearby and his wife was not present most of the day. If his physician had spoken to him in any of the preceding months or years, his affairs may have been in order with a plan in place in case something were to happen. He might have understood earlier that the services hospice could have provided would have been preferable to hospital-based life prolongation. He might have replaced his vision of hospice as "giving up" with its true function.

A beautiful hospice facility across the street from their home had a space available at the time, but because of poor communication and planning, it was not possible to transfer him there. As it happened, his last few months were confusing and difficult, with little if any communication with his doctor of 20 years. And after his death, his wife had to decipher his intentions and decide what to do with his project, his art, and his effects. At 89, this was an added stress after losing her partner, and could have been prevented if conversations about death were reasonable, practical, and expected in medicine.

The job of oncologists, geriatricians, family practitioners, and internists should be, as early as possible, to know their patients' priorities. It is possible to get to know them well, and to ask questions which might seem difficult initially but become easier with each asking. "What would you do differently if you had little time?" "What would be most important to you if medical treatment was unsuccessful or more painful than a likelihood of cure?"

My view is that the doctor's responsibility is to be very clear in communications about the extent of medical problems, possible and likely side effects of treatments, and about what might happen if their health deteriorates quickly. Most of the time there is "something more that could be done," but in many instances, doing less may allow more space and freedom for the patient to finish their lives in peace.

Questions to Ask Yourself About Dying

These questions are taken directly from Atul Gawande's book,[513] but I would like to repeat them. I suggest everyone think about these early and often. Dying isn't the best time to change anyone's life according to integrity and priorities; the best time is always today.

1. What is your understanding of your situation and its potential outcomes?
2. What are your fears and what are your hopes?
3. What are the tradeoffs you are willing to make and not willing to make?
4. What is the course of action that best serves this understanding? (Or more simply: What would a good day look like?)

Using myself as an example, my personal tradeoffs are that I am okay with needing help and medications and care to a point, but if I can't eat on my own and can't enjoy chocolate, then I'd like to be able to let go as peacefully and as comfortably as possible. I've performed CPR too many times to want it tried on me if I have more than one medical condition. I've heard similar things from doctor and nurse friends. In my experience, doctors choose very different ways of dying, when they have the choice, than many of their patients do. Changing how doctors discuss these things with their patients is the main reason for writing this chapter.

Because these kinds of changes start with us as individuals, I encourage you to contemplate your state of health and quality of life yearly, to make sure that as life changes, corresponding priority changes are taken into account. This ensures that loved ones (who may end up being asked to help you if you can't speak for yourself) understand what your wishes are, and that they are up-to-date and comfortable talking about it. Having these conversations can be difficult, but we all need to practice dealing with our fears and worries about illness and death, so that when emergencies happen, or when death approaches, our deepest wishes are respected, and instead of mostly conflict, there is peace.

Medical Pop Culture and Death Avoidance

How do we deal with a culture that is insistent that youthfulness is better than wisdom, and that fighting is the only way to live until the embarrassing defeat of death? And what should doctors do when they feel they've failed if a patient dies? Illustrative of this issue is a book that came out a short while ago by a physician who is semi-famous on the internet in the integrative medicine world. He is the type of doctor who is very sure his way is right, and the type of doctor that says things like "Fighting liver disease? Drink coffee." Not that he gives bad advice every time, and anyone advocating for a diet higher in plants is on the right track, but the title of his book is truly appalling.

Maybe by calling it *How Not to Die* he meant that sudden or unpreventable death by accident is seemingly preferable to death from chronic disease. Perhaps he meant that if one can choose behaviors that avoid chronic disease, one might contribute less to one's own death and avoid some of the sequelae of those diseases. But the fact is that the marketing message in that title is that death is bad, avoidable, and one needs his book to prevent it and ensure an extra-long life. This is plainly absurd, but it preys on our fears and cultural renunciation of death as a part of life.

The fact is that doctors like him continue to exploit our fears, usually while giving at least partially sound advice. This makes the entire matter more confusing, and causes doctors to lose credibility. This happened where I practiced in California: as integrated as my practice was, many local practitioners of alternative medicine and much of the public had little respect for physicians; many considered naturopaths or chiropractors better equipped to give good medical advice. The difference in training and knowledge didn't matter. Instead, the more science-based a doctor's understanding was, the more myopic and unhelpful he or she was perceived to be by many people in the community.

It would be helpful if individuals, alternative practitioners, and medical personnel had a better sense of Western medicine's utility, how it intersects with alternative practices, and how all of these things can be better applied to dealing with life, illness, and death. Doctors are not really here to defeat death and disease, even if that is sometimes what it looks like. Our real job is to facilitate health. Yes, that can mean an antibiotic or thyroid pill, and it can mean surgery or chemotherapy. It can even mean turning formally lethal illnesses into chronic manageable diseases, which still seems miraculous to me. But we all need to understand that Western medicine is best at responding to emergencies, and in the last century has grown to be comparatively abysmal at preventing and reversing chronic disease, caring for terminally ill patients, and dealing with aging. It is especially terrible at appreciating death and what the process of dying can teach us. Part of our cultural separation from nature is also a separation from our bodies and from natural cycles in our lives, which include death. We all need to understand these cycles better, and work with them instead of against them.

In many of these chapters we've discussed basic ways to help deal with chronic disease and improve the body's own repair mechanisms and disease-fighting capabilities. But the main element needed for doctors to implement these strategies is time. And the issue of time applies even more when working with terminally ill patients. A doctor must first have a calm, personal understanding of death in order to be comfortable discussing this inevitable outcome with patients. Then the doctor must have enough time to get to know each patient, ask the appropriate questions about priorities and wishes, and allow the patient time to think seriously and answer the questions.

Aging is no different. At each point of narrowing possibilities, as a patient's physical or mental capabilities diminish, the doctor must have time to get to know the patient and family at their new point of function. Then he or she needs to be able to hone in on the goals most important to the patient. This can mean being able to have a pet nearby, getting out into nature often, seeing family more often, to be helped to paint or sing, or to be given a responsibility like plant watering that has been proven to improve participation and interaction in assisted living facilities.

The system needs to change so that doctors can do a better job of communicating with patients, and this means we need to value the doctor-patient relationship and infuse that into the medical business model that is so dysfunctional in this country. The best presentation of these ideas I've heard was in a conversation with Atul Gawande in an *On Being* podcast interview in October 2017. I'll take the liberty of paraphrasing and adding to what Gawande said:

Primary care doctors need to be reimbursed by insurance companies (or a single-payer health system along with by Medicare or Medicaid) for the *procedure* of spending time talking to patients, whether it's about end-of-life issues, to explain disease progression or side effects of treatment, or any other time-consuming conversation, like those centered around lifestyle changes, tobacco cessation, or diet recommendations.

In our current system, specialists (doctors who went to a regular residency and then went on to do more specialized training in something like cardiology or gastroenterology) are reimbursed (paid) the most for "procedures" like heart catheterizations, colonoscopies, and even things like pap smears and skin biopsies at a far, *far* higher rate than a primary care doctor is paid for his or her time. But primary care doctors are the front lines of health care and prevention; for example, lifestyle changes, reversing early chronic diseases, and convincing people to do screening procedures and vaccinations would do more to stabilize costs and the health care economy, while saving lives at the same time, than heart catheterizations ever could.

The thing is, what doctors need most to get to know their patients well enough to be successful with these kinds of discussions is time, but time is the thing in shortest supply: doctors currently spend up to twice as long doing administrative tasks like documenting in electronic records than they do actually speaking with patients, and an average primary care visit is only 10-15 minutes long and paid at a rate that is usually around a third of what a specialist is paid.

If primary care doctors were paid comparably to specialists, more physicians would stay in primary care rather than go into subspecialties, and they might not have to work an average of 50 hours a week and burn out faster than specialists. Patients would get more time with their doctors and feel better cared for. We would be able to help people avoid many more of the 80 percent of general medical illnesses that are caused by lifestyle issues, which would reduce medication and other medical resource use, and help steer our medical system in a more sustainable direction overall. Simply by allowing doctors to bill for time spent speaking with patients about their medical issues—equating the skill and long practice that make good primary care doctors able to discuss difficult subjects with patients to the skill and practice a gastroenterologist uses to screen for colon cancer—we could quickly and rationally change our system to be much more economically efficient, patient-centered, and sustainable.

If I ever meet Dr. Gawande in person, I'd like to thank him first and foremost for this reasoned summary of the changes that need to be made.

Live as if You Are Dying, and Like You'll Live Forever

On a daily basis, many people don't trust doctors to be able to listen, to be nonjudgmental, or to know what might be best for any given patient. Medicine and science appear to be arbitrary and changeable, and since most doctors don't have time to spend on getting to know their patients well and understand where they are coming from, many patients do their best to avoid Western medicine entirely.

As with most things though, balance is crucial. It's a good idea to speak to your doctor anyway, about any illnesses you have and what the outcomes for those generally are. Ask specific questions about what would happen if you were suddenly ill or hospitalized for any reason, and make sure your physician knows exactly what interventions you do or do not want in case you were unable to communicate your wishes or became too ill to make decisions. In the current medical system, this might mean making a specific appointment to speak to your doctor about these issues, but it is well worth your time—especially if you have any medical issues already, or have parents or grandparents you are concerned about. In this case, knowledge is power, even if it is difficult to think and talk about.

Before you speak to your doctor, start by imagining what would happen if you did die suddenly, or if you become terminally ill. Imagine there isn't always a pill or something that can be done. Instead, imagine how you would feel and what would be left undone if this happened soon. Use this sort of mental space to evaluate your priorities. There is a balance, obviously, between spending all of your savings to ensure you've done everything you wanted in your life, and not dying as soon as you expected after all and finding you gave up your job and home too soon. What I do is try to look at scenarios and then pick the one in the middle that seems the best balance between responsibility and planning and living a life without any regrets. Start with, "What if I died today?" then a year from now, then five years, ten years, and twenty years. Then imagine if you were to live to be 108: What would you need to do to ensure you had a comfortable life until then? What stories would you want to be able to tell, and who would you have most wanted to spend your time with?

In this way, you will come up with a sense of your priorities. You can pick, perhaps, to focus on the 10- or 20-year goals, to ensure enough savings and prudence, but also to make sure you start integrating your life's dreams instead of putting them off for too long. Then when you discuss these topics with your doctor and your loved ones, you'll be grounded in your dreams and feel regret-free, and the conversation will more likely be a positive one. Among the patients and family members I've seen die, the things they most often truly care about that make them feel at peace are whether they lived with integrity, whether they dealt with adversity with compassion and positivity, and whether they took care of their relationships to the best of their ability.

The Value of Hospice

It takes time to get patients to understand that hospice is not "giving up," that it actually extends many patients' lives, and that it ensures the best end-of-life care possible—all according to each individual's personal wishes. Getting patients, and even their doctors, to agree to designate themselves "DNR" is difficult. Strangely difficult actually, despite doctors' knowing that CPR in the hospital rarely leads to full recovery.

This entire discussion is intended to encourage a continuing exploration of how changing our view of death can make our lives richer and more fulfilling by focusing us on what we truly believe to be important. Meditating on our own death and on our loved ones' deaths is not a morbid or depressing practice. Instead, it affords us the opportunity to appreciate life more, to be grateful for the time and health we have right at this present moment. Being familiar with and unafraid of death means that when I am able to participate in bringing a patient back and get to watch them leave the hospital after a full court press of medical science, I am uplifted and grateful to be a part of that life too.

Good Doctors Are Out There

A friend of mine, David Cumes, MD, having already trained in South Africa as a surgeon, then did a second residency in the U.S. to become board certified to practice fully here. He is an excellent surgeon and because of his reputation, before I knew him personally, he was my go-to referral for urology patients when I practiced in a small town near Santa Barbara. As I learned later, he also happens to be a shaman, or *sangoma* as it's called in South Africa.[514] He is comfortable with talking not just about death, but also discussing his philosophical framework around life and death and everything surrounding those topics. He doesn't bring his shamanic beliefs into his practice unless his patients request it, but because of this comfort with life and death, he is an expert at discussing benefits and negatives of treatments according to each patient's needs. He takes time with his patients and is much better at intuitively understanding how to communicate well with them than most surgeons I've known. Because of his pragmatic and clear approach, he is able to take both fear and unrealistic hope out of conversations with patients, focusing on truth and comfort and the patient's priorities.

Dr. Cumes also lectures at the local college and has written books about the healing power of nature and spirit. From someone who has practiced for decades in his very logical and linear surgical field, it is still highly unusual, even in a progressive town, to be able to teach yoga and meditation as well as perform his healing and spiritual practices outside of the direct cause and effect model of modern science. As he is so well respected there, he is able to be a pioneer with a firm stance in both science and the esoteric. He is an encouraging example to other physicians that this is not only possible, but it is better medicine to be able to understand with both sides of our brains and use them in concert. Meditation and the ability to let go of expectations and restrictions on what is possible helps integrate seemingly disparate ways of thinking.

Meditating on death in general helps us with our usual distorted and shortened sense of time, letting us zoom out to see a larger picture, giving us perspective that can help us live our lives more fully. Thinking realistically about death as a regular practice means that when death approaches, either quickly taking someone from us, or lingering at the doorstep for years, it no longer frightens us or triggers denial. Knowing death can catch us unawares can make us more grateful, more joyful, and more celebratory when treatments do work and patients have more time to enjoy life.

Doctors can use this more realistic approach to life and death to work through each person's priorities about how to help make life worthwhile for ourselves and for our patients. Depending on the patient's priorities, this can mean allowing time for solitude as well as for family and friends, keeping medication balanced to allow for communication as long as possible, or making sure someone's favorite food is available to taste, even if actual eating is no longer possible. It also means being open to creative solutions around nursing facility care and accommodating patients who wish to remain at home.

And of course dealing with death well means enlisting the services of hospice, social workers, and nurses, and having a team of people ready and used to assisting when difficulties arise. One of my favorite resources is Zen Hospice in San Francisco, which is not only an exceptional version of hospice but also one that connects with other organizations, hospitals, and students to train and introduce better ways of talking about death and serving the dying.[515]

There is never "nothing more we can do," there is always something lovely possible, and there is always healing available, even in someone's last moments.

APPENDIX 1

WHAT'S GOOD FOR YOU IS GOOD FOR THE PLANET: SUSTAINABLE HEALTH NUTSHELLS

Getting people to change their behavior is tricky, and there is new research showing that applying behavioral economics techniques to health care might be more effective than just suggestions or prescriptions. From addressing tendencies to externalize costs and waste, to changing how we deal with end-of-life decisions, these types of changes to how we practice medicine need community participation in discussion as well as regulatory and policy changes.[516] There is good research both on how policy changes can help people make better decisions and that they can positively affect public health, as with the ban on trans fats in New York.[517]

So many people doing great work are proving that some of the most ancient practices and principles for healing are still useful, and for some health challenges can be more effective than conventional approaches. Now we can start to find out why. The most important work, however, is done in our own lives as we start to implement these practices, so we can move forward in the best and most sustainable way possible. We can start with ourselves to create a medical paradigm that is connected to our planet instead of aloof from it, that is affordable and practical, and that empowers both patients and physicians to remove obstacles and allow the body and the planet to heal themselves as they are designed to do.

Sustainable Health Nutshells

Nutshell 1: Vote!
Pay attention to local and national politics. Vote to help small farmers and small businesses, rather than subsidizing Big Ag and tax-evading companies. Vote for improved health care for all. **Vote to help people** rather than insurance companies and pharmaceutical companies. Vote for laws and legislators who believe in environmental, economic, and social justice. **Get involved** in your community if you can, volunteering politically or otherwise. Help people get access to healthy food and health care. Support local farmers. Give your time and assistance to those more vulnerable than you.

Nutshell 2: The 4 Health Basics
Do the four "bare minimum" things that cut risks for cancer and heart disease in half (better than medications!): Quit smoking. Don't worry about being "thin" but work on getting your waist circumference down to less than 35 for women, 40 for men. Exercise a few times a week. Drink less than one alcoholic beverage a day for women, less than two for men. **No matter your age, be confident there are ways to improve your quality of health and life**. Find ways to build your health care team.

Nutshell 3: Cultivate Awareness of What Heals You
Make sure to see the forest AND the trees—help your health care provider connect the dots between your history and your current situation, and be sure to take all the complexity that your individual treatment plan needs into account. **Illnesses that came on gradually can be walked back gradually,** or at the least, slowed down or stopped; be patient and willing to experiment safely.

Nutshell 4: Regulate Your Sleep
Sleep affects blood sugar, weight, hormones, and digestion: **Go to bed around 10 p.m. and get up around 6 a.m.**, give or take an hour or so. If you have sleep disruptions, tell your doctor and see if they can be helped. If you have children that need your attention or you do shift work, 20- or 90-minute naps during the day can help with sleep deprivation (longer than 90 minutes can make you feel more tired). Weekend sleep shifts cause a system-wide stressful "jet lag" effect, so try to stay on schedule. To improve quality of sleep, stop all technology screens one to two hours before bed.

Nutshell 5: Whole Grains, Vegetables, Whole Fruits
Keep a food diary for three days, and be honest about what your favorite foods are. **Switch sugar and white flour out for whole grains**. Add servings of fresh and cooked vegetables, including beans, while taking out a few servings of meat (especially processed meat). Add a couple servings of sustainable small fish during the week. Switch out juices and sugary beverages for water and whole fruits. Cook at low temperatures, and use healthier fats like organic olive oil or (pastured) ghee. And no, you don't need to do a "cleanse."

Nutshell 6: Care for Your Ecosystem Inside and Out
Stop using antibacterial soaps and cleaning products—use plain soap. Let the kids spend lots of time playing in (pesticide/fungicide-free) dirt and with (healthy) animals. Eat a variety of plant foods (cooked, fermented, and raw), and aim for locally grown, in season produce. **Use less plastic**. Try alternatives to antibiotics when safe, using oils, teas, food, and rest to help your immune system fight off common intruders. When antibiotics are necessary, follow your doctor's instructions 100 percent. Homesteaders, do not feed your chickens antibiotic-containing feed!

Nutshell 7: Buy Local, Sustainable & Grow Your Own
Support your local sustainable farmers by buying their foods and by voting for supportive legislation to help them compete with big business. Eat more plants and **buy organic and/or sustainably farmed when you can**. Experiment with gardening, and join up with other community members to grow food to share. Help bees and other native pollinators: **plant local wildflowers** and grow everything without sprays or fungicides.

Nutshell 8: Meditate & Go Outside
Try **doing a meditation practice most days for six months**, and keep a small journal to evaluate it at the end of six months. Try a meditation app if you find it motivating. **Spend more time outside** and without your phone! Limit children's exposure to technology, and spend time in nature as a family.

Nutshell 9: Don't Sit Too Long
Change position every 30 minutes, especially if you sit for work. Set a timer, and stand, sit, walk, stretch, do a handstand—whatever it takes to keep your joints and lymphatic system moving. Try intervals! Try osteopathic manipulative treatment! Try yoga or pilates or karate! **Take breaks outside**. If you have injuries or

other limitations, don't worry, there is always something positive to do that can move lymph, increase heart rate, and improve lung capacity safely, just be sure to ask your doctor before starting something new. If you can walk or bike to work or to take care of errands, do so!

Nutshell 10: Be Patient & Willing to Adjust Your Treatment Plan
Doctors and patients both: **Be okay with being wrong or unsure, or taking a while to figure out what's wrong**. When the first or second idea doesn't work, simplify and scale back, see what might have been missed. If nothing is budging with a new treatment, **go back to basics: improve sleep first, then increase movement**, then work on food. Streamline necessary medicines and take fewer supplements; if they don't do what they've promised in three months, don't waste your money.

Nutshell 11: Think About Death as a Best-case Scenario
Make sure your family knows your wishes, and with every change in health, re-evaluate and discuss your best-case scenario and quality of life priorities. Have a medical and legal power of attorney you trust.

APPENDIX 2

DIET FADS

When I say "fad," I mean anything that's popped up in the last 50 years or so that has been marketed to make the promoter money. Many common diets have been compared and looked at long term, and none have proven to be any better than simple calorie restriction and exercise—either for weight loss or life extension.[518] [519] [520] Studies also confirm that not every "healthy food" is healthy for everyone, and that local, mostly-plant foods are best. As for people selling packages and supplements, any time a company takes a whole food, processes it, then packages it to sell it for more money, advertising that it will be the answer to everyone's health problems, it is definitely too good to be true.

Let's look at a few common diets patients have asked me about.

The "**Mediterranean Diet**" always comes out on top for many reasons.[521] As studies like "The Blue Zones" show, it may be that community and genetics *in addition to* food choices are responsible for the benefits, but the basics of the diet are solid in any case.[522] This diet revolves around fresh, home-prepared food, olive oil in moderation, local pasture-fed animals and minimal animal products overall, fresh baked bread and whole grains, and local, fresh produce, including fruits, vegetables, and lots of dark leafy greens. But the key to this diet's benefits may be more about happily preparing fresh food and enjoying it with family and friends than about each specific food chosen. Newer research shows that some people don't do well with the quantities of olive oil in the usual Mediterranean diet, so it might be good for people with Mediterranean genes, but perhaps others might do better with other types of whole foods and healthy fats, while keeping the Mediterranean cooking and social principles.

The "**Paleo**" diet is not based on good science, as preferentially eating more meat many times per day, especially processed meat (grass-fed and pastured may not be as dangerous) can increase cancer risk and is not environmentally sustainable; its carbon footprint is *enormous* compared to a vegetable-heavy diet.[523] Also, whole grains and legumes are missing from this fad, which is at best unnecessary and at worst actually harmful. Yes, eating fewer processed foods and more whole foods while increasing the amount of vegetables you eat is great, but you don't need to buy into the fad to do that.

The wisdom of avoiding **nightshades** isn't proven, and some studies show that lycopene from tomatoes and yellow and purple potatoes may actually reduce inflammation. But, as one of the more recent glycemic index studies shows, some foods like tomatoes do odd things to blood sugar in some people, so until more research comes out about other foods and other laboratory values for inflammation, we can't be sure who will have which reaction to a particular food. If it seems your allergies, arthritis, or gastrointestinal symptoms improve when you avoid nightshades, great, just make sure to replace them with other colorful vegetables.

An **elimination diet** can help iron out which specific foods do what, and it can be tedious but worthwhile for very tricky health problems. This entails scaling back your diet diversity to a very boring list of simple foods like white rice, cooked fruits, and simple vegetables, with no caffeine, onions, or garlic. An elimination diet can be helpful since when adding back foods one at a time, reactions can be noted more easily. However, it seems to work for only a very select group of patients. It can also play into disordered eating and can end up with people eating a very limited diet lacking in nutrition. I recommend giving an elimination diet a shot if you have particular health issues or think you may be allergic to a food, just remember to give it long enough—usually four to eight weeks, or until your symptoms are greatly improved. Then add foods back one or two at a time. If symptoms don't improve after eight to twelve weeks on the simplest diet, it's unlikely that food choices are contributing much to your issues.

In this same vein, the **low FODMAP** (fermentable oligosaccharides, disaccharides, monosaccharides, and polyols) diet and variations of it seem to truly benefit a select group of patients with functional intestinal disorders, but it is incredibly difficult to follow.[524] It is recommended for two to six weeks to reduce symptoms, after which patients are allowed to re-introduce foods from the list that contain non-absorbable components. I've seen people do well on this diet short and long term, but many have reactions when re-introducing foods on the list. I'm not sure it facilitates healing as much as relieves symptoms, but for some patients that is quite helpful if they've felt unwell for a long time.

Raw Food advocates are amazing chefs, but eating only raw foods makes your digestion have to work harder to obtain needed calories and nutrients. It also requires creativity, time, and processing to create textures and palatable substitutions for "usual" foods, which isn't an option available to everyone. Over time, those who practice this diet miss out on some vitamins and proteins that are more easily accessed from cooked foods and, as I've seen in my practice, immune systems and digestive systems can suffer over the long term. Raw foods are necessary and great additions to a healthy diet, but 100 percent raw (especially raw and vegan) is not helpful long term for 99 percent of the population.[525] Like the Paleo diet, this is a diet of privilege without long-term health benefits, and is not recommended.

If you are **vegan** for moral or religious reasons, great, just please make sure you get balanced proteins and enough B12, B6, D, K, K2, iron, and zinc. B12 is stored in the liver for around three to four years. Over time, if not supplementing, vegans are at risk of becoming dangerously deficient. Plant iron is abundant but is "non-heme" and harder for the body to absorb. I suggest supplementing these particular vitamins with the methylated form of B12 and folate, in case you have a genetic mutation that could curb your ability to metabolize those vitamins (which I also discuss in chapter 10).

There *is* good evidence that a very low-fat, vegan diet, along with weight loss from better diet in general, can allow your body to clear out cholesterol plaques without surgery, which is recommended if you have heart disease or are very overweight.[526][527] Given that it takes years to create plaques that lead to heart attacks and strokes, it takes years to reverse, but less time than it took to build up if you are vigilant. Since a very low-fat, vegan diet is very severe and strict, it should not be forever for most people, so make sure you are checking in with your doctor regularly. If you choose to be lacto-ovo vegetarian or pescatarian, it's much easier to make sure you get adequate nutrition. In the West, though, many vegetarians tend to overeat processed carbohydrates and cheese, so make sure to keep whole grains and vegetables at the forefront of your food choices. If you're craving cheese, you might be short on fat, salt, protein, or certain vitamins or minerals, so check out your diet's balance.

Newer versions of these diets include **Pegan** (paleo + vegan via Mark Hyman, MD) and **Valeo** (vegan + paleo via Robynne Chutkyne, MD), depending on emphasis. While I love the emphasis on vegetables and non-processed foods, I still have the same environmental issues I do with the Paleo diet where meat is emphasized so much, and especially without regard to how it is raised or cooked. I'm simply not sure the available science backs up these types of diets, particularly when they encourage eating meat from typical environmentally disastrous farms. Glycemic load is also proving to be unreliable; fear of gluten makes people avoid whole grains and legumes when they don't need to. And soy and dairy are healthy, when they are sustainably grown and grass-fed respectively, and don't need to be avoided by everyone.[528] Secondarily, eating like this (which happens to be 180 degrees opposite the "FODMAP" diet) while adding fiber supplementation might cause some people worsening gastrointestinal symptoms, and emphasizing leafy greens, without taking into account those with methylation genetic difficulties, may be problematic.

The main idea is that it is in everyone's best interest not to get fanatical about any fad diet out there, since many are misleading, and some might be hazardous. It's much easier to simply state that whole grains and whole vegetables should be the backbone of what you eat, adding fruits, fats, spices, and meats as garnish and to round out flavor and nutrition. I just don't think there needs to be a marketed name for healthy food choices, and I firmly do not believe one diet works for everyone. I would rather the simplest principles be taught to and understood by all doctors, not just famous ones, allowing doctors and patients to individualize what works best for them based on the available information.

APPENDIX 3

THE TRUTH ABOUT FASTING

There is an internet myth floating around that makes fasting sound like it's the fountain of youth. For decades, we've known that in studies on mice restricting calories increases lifespan. There are also cases of hermits and ascetic religious people living a very long time eating very, very little. There is a good amount of research that supports fasting as at least safe in certain healthy people. There are even good studies explaining exactly how fasting affects the body, and a number of suggestions are coming from these studies as to how we might want to schedule fasts to increase health and add perhaps years to our lives.

There are several caveats with fasting, though. First, we have to consider that health and metabolism are highly dependent on an individual's particular variables. So although general guidelines may eventually come out of the research being done (there aren't concrete ones yet), they need to be carefully applied to each individual. Too many people have taken the initial studies and individual cases and let their imagination run away with them. If you Google "fasting," so many results are returned that it is impossible to sift through them all, and it's very difficult to find scientific evidence backing most of them.

Add to this the Western idea that the body is "dirty" and

needs help to cleanse itself, and you get a whole industry making money from people's fear of death and dirt. Many fad diet websites offer products for purchase to perform a "juice fast," or pills and formulas to take to "detoxify" your intestines, along with testimonials from people who feel amazing after doing one of these procedures. But the problem is not the body's ability to cleanse itself. In fact, it is extraordinarily good at that naturally, especially when sleep, exercise, and diet are adequate (and not excessive). Most of the real reasons people feel great after doing a "cleanse" is that they temporarily stopped ingesting processed food, alcohol, or other drugs. After a bit of withdrawal from sugar, alcohol, and caffeine, it is normal to feel very well on little food; the body is designed to function well when hungry.[529] [530] [531] [532] [533]

But calorie restriction is tricky if one is not at optimum health, and many juice fasts and low-calorie diets not only withhold helpful nutrients that keep the intestinal microbiota fed and happy, they also add too much sugar, commonly in the form of juice, crystalline fructose, or maple syrup. These may sound "healthy," but sugar intake prevents fat burning and stops possibly helpful ketone bodies from forming when one is attempting a temporary lower-calorie diet. I also need to mention that while fragments of anecdotal evidence exist suggesting that extended periods of true fasting (drinking only calorie-free liquids) or prolonged ketosis may help with various illnesses, it is potentially dangerous, and I would never recommend something so drastic, and certainly not unless you are followed closely by a doctor at all times.

Looking at the current state of research on fasting, a few methods seem reasonable, and preliminary results from point to the possibility of long-term reductions in risks for cancer, heart disease, and diabetes. But vital to this discussion is, first, "Who is fasting safe for?" Healthy adults are the only people who should consider fasting, whether for weight loss, improved blood sugar control, or other fitness goals. Weight loss in older adults can be harmful, and for children and the ill, the body's processes are already maxed out with growing or healing, and would not benefit from the stress of a fast. Research is ongoing with obese adults ages 55–70, but for now I would recommend against any drastic measures for that age group and older. And to be clear, current research on healthy people shows absolute weight loss is the same whether from restricted calories or alternate day fasting, so fasting isn't a miraculous way to lose more weight.[534]

But for adults who have had access to food, and perhaps too much unhealthy food for several years, occasional fasting may be beneficial over time for reasons beyond weight maintenance. In the normal human metabolism, an excess of calories is stored, and an excess of sugar over time is stored as fat. Excess fat, particularly abdominal fat, can lead to inflammation and increased risk of several cancers and chronic diseases. Part of this storage issue is due to an overabundance of calories, but also because the continual input of calories, especially without the stress of intense exercise or any periods with less food, means that the body stays in an anabolic state, meaning a continual storage and "growth" state. If nutrition is inadequate, there can be a drive to eat more to hopefully bring in the missing nutrients, exacerbating the problem of overabundance of empty calories.

By contrast, fasting and intense exercise both kick in the body's breakdown or catabolic processes, and stop the continual storage of calories in favor of using what is stored. This means that when the body uses up the liver's stored glycogen during a period of fasting, or because you've just played a couple of hours of competitive soccer, it starts to tap into using the stored energy from body fat. This also allows cleanup processes to work more efficiently, getting rid of cells that aren't working optimally and repairing damage from other stresses. There is evidence that calorie restriction may be very good for brain protection and clearing the brain of toxins and plaques. In mice, fasting has been shown to offer some protection from Alzheimer's disease, but this remains to be proven in humans, though the research is promising.

A promising, very small study in the British Medical Journal shows that men with type 2 diabetes reduced their waist circumference and drastically reduced their medication in the first few weeks of one of the strictest fasting regimens.[535] Some body types and otherwise healthy patients could very well benefit from a strict fasting plan for a short time, moving to a more moderate plan when a healthier plateau is reached.

Each individual human system is a complex one with many variables. This means each individual human will benefit differently from each type of lifestyle and diet choice or change. So while there is good research to support certain types of fasting or exercise or diet, no research ever finds that the technique or idea works for everyone in the study. It is up to each person to speak with his or her doctor, to be curious about how their own body works, and to learn to listen closely and respond intelligently to its reactions. By combining knowledge of science and self-knowledge, best practices can be determined by each person. For healthy people, exercise and fewer calories will be of far more benefit than expensive vitamin products or cleansing kits. Those with more delicate health issues can still benefit by incorporating exercise and healthy diet basics into their lives at a pace that is reasonable.

Eastern Views of Fasting

It can be useful to get an understanding of the Eastern view of fasting, which is based on typical human patterns of behavior and seasonal cycles. Since ancient times, people have occasionally eaten to excess, become ill, and not completely recovered over time, or have had an affinity for foods that were poor choices for them individually. Ayurveda (Indian Medicine) has taken this into account for thousands of years, along with the fact that many people have a tendency to become ill at season change. As a result, Ayurvedic tradition schedules gentle and safe "detoxifying" procedures called *panchakarma* two to three times per year when the seasons change. These are meant to be periods of life reassessment, and include mental and emotional as well as physical healing, and always involve meditation and removal from situations of work and stress.

The most basic of these procedures involves a "fast," consisting of about 50–75 percent of one's usual intake of healthy calories, taken from only vegetables, legumes, and whole grains. Fresh foods are emphasized for best nutrition during this rejuvenation period. The timing is important, and some versions emphasize eating only two meals per day. That would encourage a period of fasting in the neighborhood of 16 hours, long enough for metabolism to switch to fat burning and to allow the benefits of fasting to be felt by the metabolism and nervous system.

The main differences between Ayurvedic and Western fasting regimes are in the specific food prescriptions, the slightly longer length of time (eight to twelve days versus five days or two days per week), and suggesting it be done once every three to four months instead of monthly or weekly. There are also variations of other types of "detoxification" extras that are often prescribed, from ritual bowel or stomach emptying, steam or dry heat to produce profuse sweating, and various procedures for skin oiling, inducing sneezing, and breathing practices.

The idea central to all of these moderate intermittent fasting ideas is that the body already cleans itself very well. The problems arise when we make poor lifestyle and diet choices, weakening our body's ability to get rid of wastes and toxins. In this sense, an Ayurvedic "cleanse" simply removes obstacles to the body's internal cleaning mechanisms while supporting the person's energy and gut microbiome with adequate nutrients and fiber during the period of lower calorie intake. Other emphases in the

Ayurvedic view include proper sleep, gentle exercise, good skin and teeth care, and the use of healthy oils. This makes sense for all of us, especially when people may be chronically compensating from lack of sleep, stress, not enough healthy food, and generally not taking care of themselves well.

If You Want to Try Fasting…

First, ask your doctor if any of these ideas are safe for you. Then, my suggestion is if you decide to undertake one of the newer fasting plans, you incorporate some of these helpful mental "cleanse" routines at the same time, renewing your mental energy and lowering emotional stress while giving your body a break. A whole-person approach makes it more of a holistic rejuvenation regimen rather than a period of simple deprivation. These regimens are meant to introduce or remind patients of healthy routines, so that when patients return to normal life, the healthy habits "stick" and continue to prevent illness.

You can start by picking one day a week, and eat a smaller lunch and much smaller dinner than usual. Make that day a day of rest and rejuvenation, meditate or pray, and spend time with family away from work, television, and internet.

Longer-Term Intermittent Fasting

If you're interested in trying one of the newer, evidence-based versions of fasting, I suggest one of the three with the best research backing so far. None have published clinical trials on humans yet, nor have long-term human studies been done. That means most of this is still conjecture and based on short-term individual case studies and blood tests from people who've given it a try. These versions have similar likely outcomes and benefits, and patient response to each type varies widely.

The first is from Dr. Valter Longo at the USC Longevity Institute, and is a very low calorie diet for three to five days per month. Since Dr. Longo has patented this version, available details are vague unless you purchase his kits. The basic idea is this: On fast day 1, eat half the normal amount of calories (so around 1,000-1,200 calories). On fast days two through five, have 35 percent or so (around 700-800 calories). The fasting day calories should be highly nutritious and whole food only, and extra water and calorie-free liquids should be taken. The rest of the month, eat a normal healthy diet based on the criteria we've already talked about.

The second version of intermittent fasting is one I've tried myself. Every week, for two days, either separate or consecutive, eat a quarter of your normal calories: around 500 for women, 600 for men. Again, the fast day foods should be highly nutritious whole foods, with plenty of calorie- and sweetener-free liquids. Ideally on the fast days, make sure 16 hours pass between dinner the night before and the first small meal, and make sure the last calorie intake of the day is at least 12 hours before breakfast the next morning. This helps the liver use up all of its glycogen stores and changes metabolic activities.

Although I didn't have access to laboratory tests, during the five weeks I tried this the first time, I did lose a couple of pounds and felt healthier. If I ever fall off the healthy wagon again for an extended period of time, I might track my progress doing the 5:2 regime with an actual scale and blood tests. Ideally, I would keep it up on a similar 6:1 schedule (six regular days, one fasting day), which is undergoing trial in the U.K. This seems to be easier to adhere to over time, and still seems to maintain the beneficial results in blood sugar and heart profile tests from the more intense 5:2 regime.

The third version is "eating in a window" or "intermittent fasting." This means eating only during a six to eight hour window during the day (and going longer without eating if you feel well).

The idea is to deplete the liver stores of sugar and burn fat for a while before eating again. The theory is that insulin release during the "fed" state makes the body hold onto calories more, while during the periods of extended fasting, fat will be burned and the body's "cleanup" mechanisms will be more efficient. During the 18 hours of fasting, it is important to not trigger the insulin response that happens when eating sugar and sugar substitutes. A friend of mine who feels wonderful on this regimen drinks coffee with oil or heavy cream for breakfast, and nothing else for hours. She has lost weight and feels healthier and clearer mentally. From what I've seen, it seems that people who do well on this plan are larger-framed with slow-burning metabolisms. Smaller-framed people and/or people who tend to get very hungry very fast and frequently have low blood sugar symptoms will likely not do well attempting this eating schedule.

So, if you are already very healthy, but are interested in improving cholesterol or blood sugar, reducing inflammation, or doing something to *possibly* extend the healthy years of your life, these three patterns may be worth a try. The last regime can be started by simply going 12 hours between dinner and breakfast and seeing how you feel. If you feel well, you can extend to 14 or 18 hours, making sure to stay hydrated during the 2–6 extra hours. This is the safest pattern to start with, even if you are on medications for diabetes, but of course you need to speak with your physician first.

Before you consider changing food habits, though, remember that if sleep and stress are your worst issues, changing your diet is unlikely to make much headway improving your overall health, so make sure to turn an eye to those first. If you have weakened digestive or immune systems, fasting may do more harm than good and may disrupt your microbiome unhelpfully. With any ongoing health issue, calorie restriction may cause problems, so please discuss **any** change in diet habits with your physician first, and if you don't feel well, discontinue immediately.

Pay particular attention to food diversity and nutrition on days you eat substantially less, and make sure you don't need to do vigorous activity and are not suffering from a cold or flu. Stop if you have any strange symptoms or aren't feeling well. Set a short time for the experiment, such as the recommended five weeks, and be flexible—evaluate your progress and slow down or continue as your doctor recommends at each check-in point. This short summary is no substitute for an individualized eating plan, as I've already made clear. I also need to emphasize again, as with the strict vegan diet for reversing heart disease, that this type of very specific eating plan is not necessary for most people.

As more study results come in, we may find that some versions of fasting a few times a year may be great for a wider subset of the population, closer to what many Eastern meditation traditions suggest. As of now though, only healthy people or those with relatively mild chronic disease issues should consider trying these plans out for longer than a few weeks, and always under a doctor's care.

"Dieting" in general has been proven to be ineffective, and most weight returns when a regular diet is resumed. But eating whole food diets and increasing the amount of plants eaten has been proven to be helpful to essentially everyone.[536] Fasting seems to be outside these criteria and the short-term benefits may persist without as many specific restrictions outside of the intermittent fasting days, which may be easier to adhere to for the length of time it takes to reverse whatever issue prompted this regimen.

ENDNOTES

1   Dan Bednarz PhD and Don Spady M.D. article 5/10 on the webpage Health After Oil. "Sustainable Medicine: An Issue Brief on Medical School Reform."

2   Trevor Thompson, PhD and Tim Ballard MD. White Paper entitled "Sustainable Medicine: good for the environment, good for people." *British Journal of General Practice* 2011 Jan 1: 61(582): 3-4.

3   K. Schroeder, T. Thompson, K. Frith, D. Pencheon. *Sustainable Healthcare*, 2012, BMJ Books.

4   London Sustainable Development Commission, 2008. "Virtuous Cycles demonstrating the benefits of a sustainable development approach."

5   John Upton, for *Salon*, 3/28/17. "Migration Crisis: Communities retreat as oceans swell, coasts erode."

6   Jim Robbins, for the *New York Times*, 7/14/12. "The Ecology of Disease."

7   Jeff Biggers, *New York Times* Op-ed, 11/20/15. "Iowa's Climate-Change Wisdom."

8   Alastair Bland *NPR's The Salt*, 12/7/15. "Carbon Farming Gets a Nod at Paris Climate Conference."

9   Charlotte Simmonds for *The Guardian*, 5/5/16. "When in drought: the California farmers who don't water their crops."

10 Roc Morin for *The Atlantic*, 10/6/14. "The Amish Farmers Reinventing Organic Agriculture."

11 Maria Finn for *Civil Eats*, 12/16/15. "The West Coast Groundfish Recovery: The Best Fish News You Haven't Heard Yet."

12 Harvard and CIA Sustainable Food recommendations called "Menus of Change. The Business of Healthy, Sustainable, Delicious Food Choices." http://www.menusofchange.org/principles-resources/moc-principles/

13   Elizabeth Grossman for *Civil Eats*, 1/6/16. "The FDA just banned these three chemicals in food. Are they the tip of the iceberg?"

14   Vincent Réquillart, *The Economist*, 11/26/15. "Small changes in climate can make a big difference to greenhouse gas emissions."

15   Damian Carrington for *The Guardian*, 10 Oct 2018. "Huge reduction in meat-eating 'essential' to avoid climate breakdown."

16   Damian Carrington for *The Guardian*. Wed 16 Jan 2019. "New plant-focused diet would 'transform' planet's future, say scientists."

17   J Cowden rev. Schwartz AE et al. The *Journal of the American Medical Association*, Pediatrics 2016 Jan 19. "Can simply providing water to students affect their weight?"

18   Avery Yale Kamila for *Portland Press Herald*, 4/13/16. "Maine Med plants seeds for doctors to focus on the health impact of food."

19   Nicola Davis for *The Guardian*. Wed 10 Oct 2018. "How to grapple with soaring world population? An answer from Botswana."

20   Misti Crane for *Ohio State University News*, 12/28/15. "River ecosystems show incredible initial recovery after dam removal."

21   James Wilt for *Vice*, 1/12/16. "There is a new climate change disaster looming in northern Canada."

22   Arthur Kleinman, *The Lancet*, Vol 375:1518-1519, 5/1/10. "Four social theories for global health."

23   Michael Hobbes for *New Republic*, 11/17/14. "Stop trying to save the world: Big ideas are destroying international development."

24   McGinnis JM, Foege WH. *JAMA* 1993 Nov 10; 270(18):2207-12. "Actual causes of death in the US" (1990) and Mokdad AH, Marks JS, et al. *JAMA* 2004 Mar 10; 291(10):1238-45. "Actual causes of death in the US, 2000."

25   Douglas A. Mata, Marco A. Ramos, et al. *JAMA* 2015; 314(22):2373-2383. "Prevalence of Depression and Depressive Symptoms Among Resident Physicians."

26   Jeffrey Brenner, MD, on the Freakonomics.com podcast. "How many doctors does it take to start a healthcare revolution?"

27   Elliott Campbell from UC Merced, 6/1/15. "Farmland mapping project indicates that more than 90 percent of US could eat food grown or raised within 100 miles of their homes, helping economy and making agriculture more sustainable."

28   Zeneng Wang, et al. *Cell*. Dec 17, 2015, Vol 163, Issue 7, p 1585-1595. "Non-lethal inhibition of gut microbial trimethylamine production for the treatment of atherosclerosis."

29   Stellar JE, et al. *Emotion*. 2015 Apr; 15(2):129-33. "Positive affect and markers of inflammation: discrete positive emotions predict lower levels of inflammatory cytokines."

30   Amit Khera, Connor Emdin, et al. *New England Journal of Medicine*. 2016 Dec 15; 375:2349-2358.

31   Aaron Carroll for the *New York Times*. 12/12/16. "The power of simple life changes to prevent heart disease."

32   C. Tomasetti, B. Vogelstein. "Variation in cancer risk among tissues can be explained by the number of stem cell divisions." *Science*. 2015 Jan 2; 347(6217): 81. (Johns Hopkins Medicine)

33   C. Tomasetti, B. Vogelstein, "Variation in cancer risk among tissues can be explained by the number of stem cell divisions." *Science*. 2015 Jan 2; 347(6217): 78-81. (Johns Hopkins Medicine)

34   Song Wu, S. Powers, et al, "Substantial contribution of extrinsic risk factors to cancer development." *Nature*. 2016 Jan 7; 529, 43-47. (Stony Brook University)

35   Aaron Carroll for the *New York Times*, 7/5/16. "Helpless to Prevent Cancer? Actually, quite a bit is in your control."

36   Mingyang Song, E. Giovannucci, "Preventable Incidence and Mortality of carcinoma associated with lifestyle factors among white adults in the US." *JAMA Oncology*. Sept 2016; 2(9):1154-1161.

37   Denise Grady for the *New York Times*. 12/19/16. "Cancer-Free: One recovery inspires another—and could help thousands."

38   http://www.edenalt.org/the-eden-alternative-in-care-communities/

39   Bob Tedeschi for STAT, Jan 4, 2018. "A physician homebuilder tries to upend the nursing home industry—and give seniors back their independence." (Update on Dr. Bill Thomas)

40   Kevin MD, 8/2015. "This is what a successful direct primary care (DPC) practice looks like" http://www.kevinmd.com/blog.

41   Burgess, J. "Improving Dementia Care with the Eden Alternative." *Nursing Times*. 2015 Mar 18024;111(12):24-5.

42   Denise Grady for the *New York Times*, 3/6/10. "Lessons at Tuba City Hospital, Run by Navajos, About Births."

43   James Surowiecki for The New Yorker, 9/22/14. "Home Free?"

44   Atul Gawande. *Being Mortal: Medicine and What Matters in the End*. Picador, 2014.

45   Kelly Rae Chi, *Nature*. 538:275-277, Oct 13, 2016.

46 *Epigenetics* 2014 Dec; 9(12):1557-69. "An integrative analysis reveals coordinated reprogramming of the epigenome and the transcriptome in human skeletal muscle after training."

47 David Auerbach for *Slate*. Jan 19, 2016. "The Theory of Everything and Then Some."

48 S. Battiston, J.D. Farmer, et al. *Science*. 19 Feb, 2016: Vol. 351, Issue 6275, 818-819. "Complexity theory and financial regulation."

49 B. Hölzel, J. Carmody, et al. *Psychiatry Research*: Neuroimaging. Vol 191 Issue 1. 30 Jan 2011, 36-43. "Mindfulness practice leads to increases in regional brain gray matter density." [8 wks MBSR]

50 C. Torgan reporting for the National Institutes of Health, June 15, 2015. "Lymphatic Vessels Discovered in Central Nervous System."

51 A. Louveau, I. Smirnov, et al. *Nature,* 523, 337-341, July 16, 2015. "Structural and functional features of central nervous system lymphatic vessels."

52 Dale Keiger for *Johns Hopkins Magazine*, Winter 2013. "Moving cancer research out of the Petri dish and into the third dimension."

53 Alan Watts. *Do You Do It or Does It Do You? How To Let the Universe Meditate You.* Sounds True audiobook, 2005.

54 Kim ES, Kawachi I, Chen Y, Kubansky LD. *JAMA Psychiatry.* Oct 1, 2017; 74(10):1039-1045. "Association between purpose in life and objective measures of physical function in older adults."

55 A-M. Chang, D. Aeschbach, et al. *Proceedings of the National Academy of Sciences of the USA*, Jan 27, 2015; vol 112 no. 4, 1232-1237. "Evening use of light-emitting eReaders negatively affects sleep, circadian timing, and next-morning alertness."

56 C. Möller-Levet, S. Archer, et al. *Proceedings of the National Academy of Sciences of the USA* (PNAS) March 19, 2013 vol 110 no 12, 1132-1141. "Effects of insufficient sleep on circadian rhythm and expression amplitude of the human blood transcriptome." [One week of insufficient sleep alters genes related to immunity, stress responses, remodeling, and regulation of gene expression.]

57 C. Liguori, A. Romigi, et al. *JAMA Neurology.* 2014;71(12):1498-1505. "Orexinergic system dysregulation, sleep impairment, and cognitive decline in Alzheimer disease."

58 R. Bernert, C. Turvey, et al. *JAMA Psychiatry.* 2014 Oct; 71(10): 1129-1137. "Association of poor subjective sleep quality with risk for death by suicide during a 10-year period. A longitudinal, population-based study of late life."

59 Patel SR, *Obesity Review.* 2009 Nov; 10 Supplement 2:61-8. "Reduced sleep as an obesity risk factor."

60 Pan A, Schernhammer ES, et al. *PLoS Medicine.* 2011 Dec; 8(12):e1001141. "Rotating night shift work and risk of type 2 diabetes: two prospective cohort studies in women."

61 F. Cappuccio, L. D'Elia, et al. *Sleep.* 2010 May 1; 33(5): 585-592. "Sleep Duration and all-cause mortality: a systematic review and meta-analysis of prospective studies."

62 S. Patel, F. Hu. *Obesity* (Silver Spring). 2008 Mar; 16(3): 643-653. "Short sleep duration and weight gain: a systematic review."

63 Gale JE, Cox HI, et al. *Journal of Biological Rhythms.* 2011 Oct; 26(5):423-33. "Disruption of circadian rhythms accelerates development of diabetes through pancreatic cell loss and dysfunction."

64 Gu F, Han J, et al. *American Journal of Preventative Medicine.* 2015 Mar; 48(3):241-52. "Total and cause-specific mortality of U.S. nurses working rotating night shifts."

65 M. Bellesi, M. Pfister-Genskow, et al. *Journal of Neuroscience.* 2013 Sep 4; 33(36): 14288-14300. "Effects of Sleep and Wake on Oligodendrocytes and Their Precursors." [Sleep, particularly REM, improves myelination of brain cells, while lack of sleep increases activity of oligodendrocytes responsible for cell death and stress response.]

66 M. Irwin, R. Olmstead, J. Carroll. *Biological Psychiatry.* July 1, 2016, vol 80, issue 1, 40-52. "Sleep disturbance, sleep duration, and inflammation: a systematic review and meta-analysis of cohort studies and experimental sleep deprivation."

67 H. Hiscock, E. Sciberras, et al. *British Medical Journal.* 2015; 350:h68. "Impact of a behavioural sleep intervention on symptoms and sleep in children with ADHD, and parental mental health: randomized controlled trial."

68 D. Blazer, K. Yaffe, et al. Committee on the Public Health Dimensions of Cognitive Aging; Board on Health Sciences Policy; Institute of Medicine. "Cognitive Aging. Progress in Understanding and Opportunities for Action." IOM suggests sufficient sleep to prevent cognitive aging.

69 L. Xie, H. Kang, M. Nedergaard, et al. *Science.* Oct 18, 2013; 342(6156). "Sleep drives metabolite clearance from the adult brain."

70 S. Da Mesquita, A. Louveau, et al. *Nature.* Aug 2018; 560 (7717): 185-191. "Functional aspects of meningeal lymphatics in ageing and Alzheimer's disease."

71 C. Torgan reporting for the *National Institutes of Health* (NIH), June 15, 2015. "Lymphatic Vessels Discovered in Central Nervous System."

72 A. Louveau, I. Smirnov, et al. *Nature.* 523, 337-341 (16 July 2015). "Structural and functional features of central nervous system lymphatic vessels."

73 Macchi MM, Bruce JN. *Frontiers in Neuroendocrinology.* 2004 Sep-Dec; 25(3-4):177-95. "Human pineal physiology and functional significance of melatonin."

74 J. Cipolla-Neto, F.G. Amaral, et al. *Journal of Pineal Research.* Vol 56, Issue 4, May 2014, pp371-381.

75 Simonneaux V, Ribelayga C. *Pharmacology Review.* 2003 Jun; 55(2):325-95. "Generation of the melatonin endocrine message in mammals: a review of the complex regulation of melatonin synthesis by norepinephrine, peptides, and other pineal transmitters."

76 Toffol E, Kalleinen N, et al. *Menopause.* May 2014;21(5):493-500. "Melatonin in perimenopausal and postmenopausal women: associations with mood, sleep, climacteric symptoms, and quality of life."

77 Barron, ML. *Biological Research for Nursing.* July 1, 2007, Vol 9, Issue 1, pp49-69. "Light exposure, melatonin secretion, and menstrual cycle parameters: An integrative review."

78 Danilenko K, Samoilova E. *PLoS Clinical Trials.* Feb 9, 2007. "Stimulatory effect of morning bright light on reproductive hormones and ovulation: Results of a controlled crossover trial."

79 Lin MC, Kripke DF, et al. *Psychiatry Research.* Aug 1990; 33(2):135-8. "Night light alters menstrual cycles."

80 Wright K, McHill A, et al. *Current Biology.* Volume 23, Issue 16, p 1554-1558, Aug 19, 2013. "Entrainment of the human circadian clock to the natural light-dark cycle."

81 J. Cipolla-Neto, F.G. Amaral, et al. *Journal of Pineal Research.* Vol 56, Issue 4, May 2014, pp371-381.

82 Liu J, Clough SJ, et al. *Annual Review of Pharmacology and Toxicology.* 2016; 56:361-83. "MT1 and MT2 Melatonin Receoptors: A therapeutic perspective."

83 C.Q. Chen, J Fichna, et al. *World Journal of Gastroenterology.* 2011 Sep 14; 17(34):3888-3898. "Distribution, function, and physiological role of melatonin in the lower gut."

84 Owino S, Contreras-Alcantara S, et al. *PLoS One.* 2016 Jan 29; 11(1):30148214. "Melatonin signaling controls the daily rhythm in blood glucose levels independent of peripheral clocks."

85 He B, Zhao Y, et al. *Journal of Pineal Research.* Apr 2016; 60(3):313-26. "The nuclear melatonin receptor RORa is a novel endogenous defender against myocardial ischemia/reperfusion injury."

86 Söderquist F, Hellström PM, Cunningham JL. *PLoS One.* Mar 30, 2015; 10(3):e0120195. "Human gastroenteropancreatic expression of melatonin and its receptors MT1 and MT2."

87 Wong RK, Yang C, et al. *Digital Discoveries in Science.* Jan 2015; 60(1):186-94. "Melatonin regulation as a possible mechanism for probiotic (VSL#3) in irritable bowel syndrome: a randomized double-blinded placebo study."

88 Gupta YK, Gupta M, Kohli K. *Indian Journal of Physiology and Pharmacology.* Oct 2003; 47(4):373-86. "Neuroprotective role of melatonin in oxidative stress vulnerable brain."

89 Mahlberg R, Walther S, et al. *Neurobiology of Aging.* Feb 2008; 29(2):203-9. "Pineal calcification in Alzheimer's disease: an in vivo study using computed tomography."

90 Gupta YK, Gupta M, Kohli K. *Indian Journal of Physiology and Pharmacology.* Oct 2003; 47(4):373-86. "Neuroprotective role of melatonin in oxidative stress vulnerable brain."

91 R. Nagendra, N. Maruthai, B. Kutty. *Frontiers in Neurology.* 2012; 3:54. "Meditation and its regulatory role on sleep."

92 Tooley GA, Armstrong SM, et al. *Biological Psychology.* May 2000; 53(1):69-78. "Acute increases in night-time plasma melatonin levels following a period of meditation."

93 Westrin A, Lam RW. *Annals of Clinical Psychiatry.* 2007 Oct-Dec; 19(4):239-46. "Seasonal affective disorder: a clinical update."

94 *Epigenetics.* 2014 Dec; 9(12):1557-69. "An integrative analysis reveals coordinated reprogramming of the epigenome and the transcriptome in human skeletal muscle after training."

95 M. Irwin, R. Olmstead, J. Carroll. *Biological Psychiatry.* July 1, 2016, vol 80, issue 1, 40-52. "Sleep disturbance, sleep duration, and inflammation: a systematic review and meta-analysis of cohort studies and experimental sleep deprivation."

96   H. Hiscock, E. Sciberras, et al. *British Medical Journal.* 2015; 350:h68. "Impact of a behavioural sleep intervention on symptoms and sleep in children with ADHD, and parental mental health: randomized controlled trial."

97   D. Blazer, K. Yaffe, et al. Committee on the Public Health Dimensions of Cognitive Aging; Board on Health Sciences Policy; Institute of Medicine. "Cognitive Aging. Progress in Understanding and Opportunities for Action." IOM suggests sufficient sleep to prevent cognitive aging.

98   C. Möller-Levet, S. Archer, et al. *Proceedings of the National Academy of Sciences of the USA* (PNAS) March 19, 2013, Vol 110, No 12, 1132-1141. "Effects of insufficient sleep on circadian rhythm and expression amplitude of the human blood transcriptome." [One week of insufficient sleep alters genes related to immunity, stress responses, remodeling, and regulation of gene expression.]

99   M. Bellesi, M. Pfister-Genskow, et al. *Journal of Neuroscience.* 2013 Sep 4; 33(36): 14288-14300. "Effects of Sleep and Wake on Oligodendrocytes and Their Precursors." [Sleep, particularly REM, improves myelination of brain cells, while lack of sleep increases activity of oligodendrocytes responsible for cell death and stress response.]

100 Mortimer JA, Ding D, et al. *Journal of Alzheimers Disease.* 2012; 30(4):757-66. "Changes in brain volume and cognition in a randomized trial of exercise and social interaction in a community-based sample of non-demented Chinese elders."

101 Colombe SJ, Erickson KI, et al. *Journal of Geronology, Biological Sciences and Medical Sciences* Series A. 2006 Nov; 61(11):1166-70. "Aerobic exercise training increases brain volume in aging humans."

102 Uusi-Rasi K, Patil R. et al. *JAMA Internal Medicine.* May 2015; 175(5):703-11. "Exercise and vitamin D in fall prevention among older women: a randomized clinical trial."

103 C. Lunghi, Sale A. *Current Biology.* Volume 25, Issue 23, pR1122-3, 7 Dec 2015. "A cycling lane for brain rewiring."

104 Olga Khazan for *The Atlantic.* March 24, 2014. "For Depression, Prescribing Exercise Before Medication."

105 Kripke DF, Langer RD, Kline LE. *BMJ Open.* 2012; 2:e000850. "Hypnotics' association with mortality or cancer: a matched cohort study." Less than 18 sleep aids per year (including Benadryl) doubles

risk of death, more increases risk by 5 times and is associated with increased cancer risk.

Rev article in F1000 Research by same, Kripke, May 2016. https:// www.ncbi.nlm.nih.gov/pmc/articles/PMC4890308/

106 B. Sivertsen, I. Madsen, et al. *Drugs Real World Outcomes.* 2015 Jun; 2(2): 123-128. "Use of sleep medications and mortality: The Hordaland Health Study."

107 S. Billioti de Gage, Y. Moride, et al. *British Medical Journal.* 2014; 349:g5205. "Benzodiazepine use and risk of Alzheimer's disease: case-control study."

108 Buxton OM, Ellenbogen JM, et al. *Annals of Internal Medicine.* Aug 7, 2012; 157(3):170-9. "Sleep disruption due to hospital noises: a prospective evaluation."

109 Jaiswal SJ, Garcia S, Owens RL. *Journal of Hospital Medicine.* 2017 Oct; 12(10):798-804. "Sound and light levels are similarly disruptive in ICU and non-ICU wards."

110 Mata D, Ramos M, et al. *JAMA.*

111 Y. Hu, A. Shmygelska, et al. *Nature Communications.* 7, article number 10448, 2 Feb 2016. "GWAS of 89,283 individuals identifies genetic variants associated with self-reporting of being a morning person."

112 Bartick M, Thai X, et al. *Journal of Hospital Medicine.* 18 Sept, 2009; 5: E20-E24. "Decrease in as-needed sedative use by limiting nighttime sleep disruptions from hospital staff."

113 Bartick M, Thai X, et al. *Journal of Hospital Medicine.* 18 Sept, 2009; 5: E20-E24. "Decrease in as-needed sedative use by limiting nighttime sleep disruptions from hospital staff."

114 National Institute of Neurological Disorders and Stroke. "Brain Basics: Understanding Sleep." Patient and caregiver education online. http:// www.ninds.nih.gov/disorders/brain_basics/understanding_sleep.htm

115 K Reid, G Santostasi, et al. *PLoS One.* April 2, 2014. https://doi. org/10.1371/journal.pone.0092251 "Timing and Intensity of Light Correlate with Body Weight in Adults."

116 A Williamson, A Feyer. *Occupational Environmental Medicine.* 2000 Oct; 57(10): 649-655. "Moderate sleep deprivation produces impairments in cognitive and motor performance equivalent to legally prescribed levels of alcohol intoxication."

117 Thompson Coon J, Boddy K, et al. *Environmental Science and Technology.* 2011 Mar 1; 45(5):1761-72. "Does participating in physical activity in outdoor natural environments have a greater effect

on physical and mental wellbeing than physical activity indoors? A systematic review."

118 Richard Mitchell for University of Glasgow (published in *University News*, 20 June, 2012). "Regular exercise in natural environments halves the risk of poor mental health."

119 J Barton, J Pretty. *Environmental Science and Technology.* 2010, 44(10), pp3947-3955. "What is the best dose of nature and green exercise for improving mental health? A multi-study analysis."

120 Kripke DF, Langer RD, Kline LE. BMJ *Open.* 2012; 2:e000850. "Hypnotics' association with mortality or cancer: a matched cohort study." Less than 18 sleep aids per year (including Benadryl) doubles risk of death, more increases risk by 5 times and is associated with increased cancer risk. Rev article in F1000. Research by same, Kripke, May 2016. https://www.ncbi.nlm.nih.gov/pmc/articles/PMC4890308/

121 Simon Parkin for *The Guardian.* 14 Sep, 2018. "Finally, a cure for insomnia?"

122 T Bridger. *Paediatrics Child Health.* 2009 Mar; 14(3): 177-182. "Childhood obesity and cardiovascular disease."

123 *The Economist* daily chart, Nov 14, 2016. "Diabetes is no longer a rich-world disease."

124 T Bridger. *Paediatrics Child Health.* 2009 Mar; 14(3): 177-182. "Childhood obesity and cardiovascular disease."

125 *The Economist* daily chart, Nov 14, 2016. "Diabetes is no longer a rich-world disease."

126 C-W Cheng, G Adams, et al. *Cell Stem Cell.* Volume 14, Issue 6, p 810-823, 5 June 2014. "Prolonged fasting reduces IGF-1/PKA to promote hematopoietic-stem-cell-based regeneration and reverse immunosuppression."

127 S Brandhorst, I Y Choi, et al. *Cell Metabolism.* Volume 22, Issue 1, p86-99, 7 July 2015. "A periodic diet that mimics fasting, promotes multi-system regeneration, enhanced cognitive performance, and healthspan."

128 D Zeevi, T Korem et al. *Cell.* Volume 163, Issue 5, p1079-1094, 19 Nov 2015. "Personalized Nutrition by Prediction of Glycemic Responses."

129 SM O'Mahony, G Clarke, et al. *Behavioural Brain Research.* Volume 277, 15 Jan 2015, pp32-48. "Serotonin, tryptophan metabolism and the brain-gut microbiome axis."

130 S Wu, A Liao, et al. *American Journal of Pathology.* 2010 Aug; 177(2): 686-697. "Vitamin D receptor negatively regulates bacterial-stimulated NF-kB activity in the intestine."

131 N Ly, A Litonjua, et al. *Journal of Allergy and Clinical Immunology.* 2011 May; 127(5): 1087-1094. "Gut microbiota, probiotics, and vitamin D: interrelated exposures influencing allergy, asthma, and obesity?"

132 Laparra JM, Sanz Y. *Pharmacology Research.* 2010 Mar; 61(3):219-25. "Interactions of gut microbiota with functional food components and nutraceuticals."

133 L Galland. *Journal of Medicinal Food.* 2014 Dec 1; 17(12): 1261-1272. "The Gut Microbiome and the Brain."

134 S Collins, Z Kassam, P Bercik. *Current Opinion in Microbiology.* Volume 16, Issue 3, June 2013, pp 240-245. "The adoptive transfer of behavioral phenotype via the intestinal microbiota: experimental evidence and clinical implications."

135 K Tillisch, J Labus, et al. *Gastroenterology.* June 2013, Vol 144, Issue 7, pp1394-1401.e4. "Consumption of fermented milk product with probiotic modulates brain activity."

136 Peter Andrey Smith for the *New York Times*, June 23, 2015. "Can the bacteria in your gut explain your mood?"

137 The DASH diet is a dietary pattern promoted by the U.S.-based National Heart, Lung, and Blood Institute to prevent and control hypertension.

138 Diets high in fish are associated with better health outcomes and likely lower inflammation, however, eating too much fish packed in oil may overwhelm some people's gall bladder and/or pancreatic capacity, and many fisheries are overharvested to the point of collapse. My advice is to stick to sustainably-caught small fish like sardines packed in water. If you'd like to try adding fish to your diet, try one serving two to three times a week.

139 D Zeevi, T Korem, et al. *Cell.* Volume 163, Issue 5, P1079-1094, 19 Nov, 2015. "Personalized nutrition by prediction of glycemic responses."

140 Kate Murphy for the *New York Times.* Well Blog. Jan 11, 2016. "A personalized diet, better suited to you."

141 M Springman, HC Godfray, et al. Proceedings of the National Academy of Sciences. April 12, 2016, Vol 113 No 15, p 4146-4151. "Analysis and valuation of the health and climate change cobenefits of dietary change."

142 DL Katz, S Meller. *Annual Review of Public Health.* Vol. 35:83-103. March 2014. "Can we say what diet is best for health?"

143 R Wilder. *JAMA.* 1956; 162(17):1539-1541. "A brief history of the enrichment of flour and bread."

144 Tom Philpott for *Mother Jones.* Feb 3, 2016. "WTF happened to Golden Rice?"

145 H Wu, A Flint, et al. *JAMA Internal Medicine.* March 2015; 175(3):373-384. "Association between dietary whole grain intake and the risk of mortality. Two large prospective studies in US men and women."

146 D Jenkins, C Kendall, et al. *JAMA Archives of Internal Medicine.* Nov 2012; 172(21):1653-1660. "Effect of legumes as part of a low glycemic index diet on glycemic control and cardiovascular risk factors in type 2 diabetes mellitus. A randomized controlled trial."

147 T Fung, F Hu, et al. *American Journal of Clinical Nutrition.* Sept 2002, Vol. 76, No. 3, pp535-540. "Whole-grain intake and the risk of type 2 diabetes: a prospective study in men."

148 Aune D, Keum N, et al. British Medical Journal. 2016 Jun 14; 353:i2716. "Whole grain consumption and risk of cardiovascular disease, cancer, and all-cause and cause-specific mortality: a systematic review and dose-response meta-analysis of prospective studies."

149 Chan JM, Wang F, Holly EA. *Cancer Causes Control.* 2007 Dec; 18(10):1153-67. "Pancreatic cancer, animal protein and dietary fat in a population-based study, SF Bay Area, CA."

150 Chan JM, Wang F, Holly EA. *American Journal of Epidemiology.* 2007 Nov 15; 166(10):1174-85. "Whole grains and risk of pancreatic cancer in a large population-based case-control study in the SF Bay Area, CA."

151 Venn BJ, Mann JI. *European Journal of Clinical Nutrition.* 2004 Nov; 58(11):1443-61. "Cereal grains, legumes and diabetes."

152 Liu S, Willett WC, et al. *American Journal of Clinical Nutrition.* 2003 Nov; 78(5):920-7. "Relation between changes in intakes of dietary fiber and grain products and changes in weight and development of obesity among middle-aged women."

153 Jo Robinson for the *New York Times.* May 25, 2013. "Breeding the Nutrition Out of Our Food."

154 Michele Bertelli and Javier Sauras for *Al Jazeera.* 25 July, 2013. "Quinoa boom a mixed blessing for bolivians."

155 Jenkins, D.J., et al. *Metabolism*. April 2001; 50(4): p. 494-503. "Effect of a very-high-fiber vegetable, fruit, and nut diet on serum lipids and colonic function."

156 D Ornish, SE Brown, et al. *The Lancet*. 21 July, 1990. Vol 336, No. 8708, p129-133. "Can lifestyle changes reverse coronary heart disease? The Lifestyle Heart Trial."

157 Shai I, Spense JD, et al. *Circulation*. 2010 Mar 16; 121(10):1200-8. "Dietary intervention to reverse carotid atherosclerosis."

158 K Milton. *Nutrition*. 1999 Jun; 15(6):488-498. "Nutritional characteristics of wild primate foods: do the diets of our closest living relatives have lessons for us?"

159 Fonseca-Azevedo K, Herculano-Houzel S. *PNAS USA*. 2012 Nov 6; 109(45):18571-6. "Metabolic constraint imposes tradeoff between body size and number of brain neurons in human evolution."

160 J Zou, B Chassaing, et al. *Cell Host Microbe*. 2018 Jan 10; 23(1):41-53. e4. "Fiber-mediated nourishment of gut microbiota protects against diet-induced obesity by restoring IL-22-mediated colonic health."

161 X Wang, Y Ouyang, et al. *British Medical Journal*. 2014; 349:g4490. "Fruit and vegetable consumption and mortality from all causes, cardiovascular disease, and cancer: systematic review and dose-response meta-analysis of prospective cohort studies."

162 Carter P, Gray LJ, et al. *British Medical Journal*. 2010 Aug 18; 341:c4229. "Fruit and vegetable intake and incidence of type 2 diabetes mellitus: systematic review and meta-analysis."

163 Joshipura KJ, Hu FB, et al. *Annals of Internal Medicine*. 2001 Jun 19; 134(12):1106-14. "The effect of fruit and vegetable intake on risk for coronary heart disease."

164 Bazzano LA, He J, et al. *American Journal of Clinical Nutrition*. 2002 Jul; 76(1):93-9. "Fruit and vegetable intake and risk of cardiovascular disease in US adults: the first national health and nutrition examination survey epidemiologic follow-up study."

165 Jo Robinson. *Eating on the Wild Side*. Little, Brown and Company; 1st edition June 4, 2013.

166 J Barrett. *Environmental Health Perspectives*. 2006 Jun; 114(6): A352-A358. "The science of soy: What do we really know?"

167 Jo Robinson, *Eating on the Wild Side*. Little, Brown and Company; 1st edition June 4, 2013.

168 Daphne Miller, M.D. *The Jungle Effect*. William Morrow, 2008.

169 Alice Walton for *Forbes*. May 7, 2015. "A Healthy Diet May Help The Brain Age Well, Study Finds." (cited A Smyth, M Dehghan, et al. *Neurology*. 2015 Jun 2; 84(22): 2258-2265. "Healthy eating and reduced risk of cognitive decline."

170 L Hunter Lovins in *The Guardian Sustainable Business*. 19 August 2014. "Why George Monbiot is wrong: grazing livestock can save the world."

171 George Monbiot in *The Guardian*. 22 December, 2015. "Warning: your festive meal could be more damaging than a long-haul flight."

172 Twilight Greenaway in *Civil Eats*. 4-12-16. Interview with Patrick Holden, director of the Sustainable Food Trust in the UK. "In search of the true cost of industrial meat."

173 World Health Organization Q&A on carcinogenicity of the consumption of red meat and processed meat. Oct 2-15. http://www.who.int/features/qa/cancer-red-meat/en/

174 Aaron Carroll for the *New York Times*. March 30, 2015. "Red meat is not the enemy." M.S.L.J. for *The Economist*. April 19, 2016. "Why eating more vegetables is good for the environment."

175 Sara Reardon for *Nature*. 12 June, 2017. "Resistance to last-ditch antibiotic has spread farther than anticipated." https://www.nature.com/news/resistance-to-last-ditch-antibiotic-has-spread-farther-than-anticipated-1.22140.

176 Sept 11, 2018 Lancet M. Dehghan, A Mente, et al. epub ahead of print, pubmed link: https://www.ncbi.nlm.nih.gov/pubmed/30217460

177 Jerry Adler for *Smithsonian*. June 2013. "Why Fire Makes Us Human."

178 Michael Pollan youtube video on cooking: https://www.youtube.com/watch?v=N7Ty8HoIEEg

179 D Mozaffarian, E Rimm. *JAMA*. 2006; 296(15):1885-1889. "Fish intake, contaminants, and human health."

180 Jason Mark in *Scientific American*. Aug 14, 2011. "Myths: Busted—Clearing Up the Misunderstandings About Organic Farming."

181 Michael Hamm in *The Guardian*. 10 April, 2015. "The buzz around indoor farms and artificial lighting makes no sense."

182 Alastair Bland in *NPR*'s *The Salt*. Dec 7, 2015. "Carbon Farming Gets a Nod at Paris Climate Conference."

183 Jeff Biggers in the *New York Times*. Nov 20, 2015. "Iowa's Climate-Change Wisdom."

184 Environmental Working Group's "Dirty Dozen" and "Clean 15" lists. www.ewg.org/foodnews/clean_fifteen_list.php and www.ewg.org/foodnews/dirty_dozen_list.php

185 Mitchell AE, Hong YJ, et al. *Journal of Agriculture and Food Chemistry.* 2007 Jul 25; 55(15):6154-9. "Ten-year comparison of the influence of organic and conventional crop management practices on the content of flavonoids in tomatoes."

186 Consumer Reports produce guidelines: "Eat the peach not the pesticide." https://www.consumerreports.org/cro/health/natural-health/pesticides/index.htm

187 Dan Buettner. *National Geographic.* April 2015. "The Blue Zones Solution: Eating and Living Like the World's Healthiest People."

188 Holt-Lunstad J, Smith TB, Layton JB. *PLoS Medicine.* 2010 Jul 27; 7(7):e1000316. "Social relationships and mortality risk: a meta-analytic review."

189 David Montgomery and Anne Biklé in *Nautilus.* Dec 10, 2015. "What your microbiome wants for dinner."

190 Y Furusawa, Y Obata, et al. *Nature.* 19 December, 2013; 504, 446-450. "Commensal microbe-derived butyrate induces the differentiation of colonic regulatory T cells."

191 M Dominguez-Bello, K De Jesus-Laboy, et al. *Nature Medicine.* 2016 Mar; 22(3): 250-253. "Partial restoration of the microbiota of cesarean-born infants via vaginal microbial transfer."

192 Josef Neu, J Rushing. *Clinical Perinatology.* 2011 Jun; 38(2): 321-331. "Cesarean versus vaginal delivery: long term infant outcomes and the hygiene hypothesis."

193 S Huh, S Rifas-Shiman, et al. *British Medical Journal* Archives of Disease in Childhood. 2012; 97:610-616. "Delivery by caesarian section and risk of obesity in preschool age children: a prospective cohort study."

194 Rutayisire E, Huang K, et al. *BMC Gastroenterology.* 2016 Jul 30; 16(1):86. "The mode of delivery affects the diversity and colonization pattern of the gut microbiota during the first year of infants' life: a systematic review."

195 C Guinane, P Cotter. *Therapeutic Advances in Gastroenterology.* 2013 Jul; 6(4): 295-308. "Role of the gut microbiota in health and chronic gastrointestinal disease: understanding a hidden metabolic organ."

196 D Zeevi, T Korem et al. *Cell.* 19 Nov, 2015; Volume 163, Issue 5, p1079-1094. "Personalized Nutrition by Prediction of Glycemic Responses."

197 M Dominguez-Bello, K De Jesus-Laboy, et al. *Nature Medicine.* 2016 Mar; 22(3): 250-253. "Partial restoration of the microbiota of cesarean-born infants via vaginal microbial transfer."

198 Jašarević E, Howerton CL, et al. *Endocrinology.* 2015 Sep; 156(9):3265-76. "Alterations in the vaginal microbiome by maternal stress are associated with reprogramming of the offspring gut and brain."

199 DiGiulio DB, Callahan BJ, et al. *Proceedings of the National Academy of Sciences.* 2015 Sep 1; 112(35):11060-5. "Temporal and special variation of the human microbiota during pregnancy."

200 Urbaniak C, Angelini M, et al. *Microbiome.* 2016 Jan 6;4:1. "Human milk microbiota profiles in relation to birthing method, gestation and infant gender."

201 Paramasivam K, Michie C, et al. *International Journal of Fertility and Womens Medicine.* 2006 Sep-Oct;51(5):208-17. "Human breast milk immunology: a review."

202 Brandtzaeg P. *Journal of Pediatrics.* 2010 Feb;156(2 Suppl):S8-15. "The mucosal immune system and its integratin with the mammary glands."

203 F Hassiotou, A Hepworth, et al. *Clinical & Translational Immunology.* 2013 Apr; 2(4): e3. "Maternal and infant infections stimulate a rapid leukocyte response in breastmilk."

204 S. El Aidy, T Dinan, J. Cryan. *Frontiers in Microbiology.* 2014; 5: 146. "Immune modulation of the brain-gut-microbe axis."

205 M Dominguez-Bello, K De Jesus-Laboy, et al. *Nature Medicine.* 2016 Mar; 22(3): 250-253. "Partial restoration of the microbiota of cesarean-born infants via vaginal microbial transfer."

206 M Dominguez-Bello, K De Jesus-Laboy, et al. *Nature Medicine.* 2016 Mar; 22(3): 250-253. "Partial restoration of the microbiota of cesarean-born infants via vaginal microbial transfer."

207 C de Lara, A Noble. *Biologics.* 2007 Jun; 1(2): 139-150. "Dishing the dirt on asthma: What we can learn from poor hygiene."

208 C de Lara, A Noble. *Biologics.* 2007 Jun; 1(2): 139-150. "Dishing the dirt on asthma: What we can learn from poor hygiene."

209 Olszak T, An D, et al. *Science.* 2012 Apr 27;336(6080):489-93. "Microbial exposure during early life has persistent effects on natural killer T cell function."

210 S Kinra, G Davey Smith, et al. *Thorax.* 2006 Jan; 61(1): 48-53. "Association between sibship size and allergic diseases in the Glasgow Alumni Study."

211 Adler A, Tager I, Quintero DR. *Journal of Allergy and Clinical Immunology.* 2005 Jan;115(1):67-73. "Decreased prevalence of asthma among farm-reared children compared with those who are rural but not farm-reared."

212 O Koren, J Goodrich, et al. *Cell.* 2012 Aug 3; 150(3): 470-480. "Host remodeling of the gut microbiome and metabolic changes during pregnancy."

213 L Rankin, M Girard-Madoux, et al. *Nature Immunology.* 2016 vol 17, p179-186. "Complementarity and redundancy of IL-22-producing innate lymphoid cells."

214 Dethlefsen L, Huse S, et al. *PLoS Biology.* 2008 Nov 18;6(11):e280. "The pervasive effects of an antibiotic on the human gut microbiota, as revealed by deep 16S rRNA sequencing."

215 Pérez-Cobas AE, Gosalbes MJ, et al. *Gut.* 2013;62:1591-1601. "Gut microbiota disturbance during antibiotic therapy: a multi-omic approach."

216 T Ichinohe, I Pang, et al. *PNAS.* 2011 Mar 29; 108(13): 5354-5359. "Microbiota regulates immune defense against respiratory tract influenza A virus infection."

217 Ungaro R, Bernstein CN, et al. *American Journal of Gastroenterology.* 2014 Nov;109(11):1728-38. "Antibiotics associated with increased risk of new-onset Crohn's disease but not ulcerative colitis: a meta-analysis."

218 K Blumenthal, I Youngster, et al. *Journal of Allergy and Clinical Immunology.* 2015 Nov; 136(5): 1288-1294.e1. "Peripheral blood eosinophilia and hypersensitivity reactions among patients receiving outpatient parenteral antibiotics."

219 T Ichinohe, I Pang, et al. *PNAS.* 2011 Mar 29; 108(13): 5354-5359. "Microbiota regulates immune defense against respiratory tract influenza A virus infection."

220 B Zhang, B Chassaing, et al. *Science.* 2014 Nov 14. Vol 346, Issue 6211, pp 861-865. "Prevention and cure of rotavirus infection via TLR5/ NLRC4-mediated production of IL-22 and IL-18."

221 Ungaro R, Bernstein CN, et al. *American Journal of Gastroenterology.* 2014 Nov;109(11):1728-38. "Antibiotics associated with increased risk of new-onset Crohn's disease but not ulcerative colitis: a meta-analysis."

222 Jane Brody for the *New York Times*. Sept 10, 2012. "Popular antibiotics may carry serious side effects."

223 A Demirjian, G Sanchez, et al. *CDC Morbidity and Mortality Weekly Report*. August 21, 2015 / 64(32);871-873. "CDC Grand Rounds; Getting Smart About Antibiotics."

224 A Demirjian, G Sanchez, et al. *CDC Morbidity and Mortality Weekly Report*. August 21, 2015 / 64(32);871-873. "CDC Grand Rounds; Getting Smart About Antibiotics."

225 US Dept of Health and Human Services CDC official statement 2013. "Antibiotic Resistance Threats in the United States, 2013." http://www.cdc.gov/drugresistance/threat-report-2013/pdf/ar-threats-2013-508.pdf

226 US Dept of Health and Human Services CDC official statement 2013. "Antibiotic Resistance Threats in the United States, 2013." http://www.cdc.gov/drugresistance/threat-report-2013/pdf/ar-threats-2013-508.pdf

227 E Chelossi, L Vezzulli, et al. *Aquaculture*. Vol 219, Issues 1-4, pp 83-97, 2 Apr 2003. "Antibiotic resistance of benthic bacteria in fish-farm and control sediments of the Western Mediterranean."

228 Shah SQ, Cabello FC, et al. *Environmental Microbiology*. 2014 May;16(5):1310-20. "Antimicrobial resistance and antimicrobial resistance genes in marine bacteria from salmon aquaculture and non-aquaculture sites."

229 BS Schwartz, J Pollak, et al. *International Journal of Obesity*. 2016, vol 40, 615-621. "Antibiotic use and childhood body mass index trajectory."

230 J Savage, E Matsui, et al. *Journal of Allergy and Clinical Immunology*. 2012 Aug; 130(2): 453-60.e7. "Urinary levels of triclosan and parabens are associated with aeroallergen and food sensitization."

231 M Dinwiddie, P Terry, J Chen. *International Journal of Environmental Research and Public Health*. 2014 Feb; 11(2): 2209-2217. "Recent Evidence Regarding Triclosan and Cancer Risk."

232 A Zota, C Phillips, S Mitro. *Environmental Health Perspectives*. 2016 Oct; 124(10): 1521-1528. "Recent fast food consumption and bisphenol A and phthalates exposures among the U.S. population in NHANES, 2003-2010."

233 Boberg J, Taxvig C, et al. *Reproductive Toxicology*. 2010 Sep;30(2):301-12. "Possible endocrine disrupting effects of parabens and their metabolites."

234 A Calafat, X Ye, et al. *Environmental Health Perspectives*. 2010 May; 118(5): 679-685. "Urinary concentrations of four parabens in the U.S. population: NHANES 2005-2006."

235 Halden RU. *Environment, Science, and Technology*. 2014 Apr 1;48(7):3603-11. "On the need and speed of regulating triclosan and triclocarban in the United States."

236 Nicholas Kristof for the *New York Times*. Nov 28, 2015. "Contaminating our bodies with everyday products."

237 Shehata AA, Schrödl W, et al. *Current Microbiology*. 2013 Apr;66(4):350-8. "The effect of glyphosate on potential pathogens and beneficial members of poultry microbiota in vitro."

238 A Aris, S Leblanc. *Reproductive Toxicology*. 2011 May;31(4):528-33. "Maternal and fetal exposure to pesticides associated to genetically modified foods in eastern townships of Quebec, Canada."

239 O Koren, J Goodrich, et al. *Cell*. 2012 Aug 3; 150(3): 470-480. "Host remodeling of the gut microbiome and metabolic changes during pregnancy."

240 Fuhrman BJ, Feigelson HS, et al. *Journal of Clinical Endocrinology and Metabolism*. 2014 Dec; 99(12):4632-40. "Associations of the fecal microbiome with urinary estrogens and estrogen metabolites in postmenopausal women."

241 E Dinsdale, W Ward. *Nutrients*. 2010 Nov;2(11):1156-1187. "Early exposure to soy isoflavones and effects on reproductive health: a review of human and animal studies."

242 Messina M. *American Journal of Clinical Nutrition*. 2014 Jul;100 Suppl 1:423S-30S. "Soy foods, isoflavones, and the health of postmenopausal women."

243 J Markle, D Frank, et al. *Science*. 1 Mar 2013, vol 339, issue 6123, pp. 1084-1088. "Sex differences in the gut microbiome drive hormone-dependent regulation of autoimmunity."

244 Linskens RK, Huijsdens XW, et al. *Scandinavian Journal of Gastroenterology Supplement*. 2001;(234):29-40. "The bacterial flora in inflammatory bowel disease: current insights in pathogenesis and influence of antibiotics and probiotics."

245 García Rodríguez LA, Ruigómez A, Panés J. *Gastroenterology*. 2006 May;130(6):1588-94. "Acute gastroenteritis is followed by an increased risk of inflammatory bowel disease."

246 Ruigómez A, García Rodríguez LA, Panés J. *Clinical Gastroenterology and Hepatology*. 2007 Apr;5(4):465-9. "Risk of irritable bowel

syndrome after an episode of bacterial gastroenteritis in general practice: influence of comorbidities."

247 N Molodecky, G Kaplan. *Gastroenterology and Hepatology.* 2010 May; 6(5): 339-346. "Environmental risk factors for inflammatory bowel disease."

248 Liu J, Hou X. *Gastroenterology and Hepatology.* 2011 Apr;26 Suppl 3:88-93. "A review of the irritable bowel syndrome investigation on epidemiology pathogenesis and pathophysiology in China."

249 Kerckhoffs AP, Akkermans LM, et al. *Digital Discussions in Science.* 2010 Mar;55(3):716-23. "Intestinal permeability in irritable bowel syndrome patients: effects of NSAIDs"

250 Wang Z, Klipfell E, et al. *Nature.* 2011 Apr 7;472(7341):57-63. "Gut flora metabolism of phosphatidylcholine promotes cardiovascular disease."

251 Christakis NA, Fowler JH. *NEJM.* 2007 Jul 26;357(4):370-9. "The spread of obesity in a large social network over 32 years."

252 *Radiolab* episode: "Parasites" http://www.radiolab.org/story/91689-parasites/.

253 House PK, Vyas A, Sapolsky R. *PLoS One.* 2011;6(8):e23277. "Predator cat odors activate sexual arousal pathways in brains of Toxoplasma gondii infected rats."

254 L Galland. *Journal of Medicinal Food.* 2014 Dec 1; 17(12): 1261-1272. "The Gut Microbiome and the Brain."

255 S Collins, Z Kassam, P Bercik. *Current Opinion in Microbiology.* Volume 16, Issue 3, June 2013, pp 240-245. "The adoptive transfer of behavioral phenotype via the intestinal microbiota: experimental evidence and clinical implications."

256 K Tillisch, J Labus, et al. *Gastroenterology.* June 2013, Vol 144, Issue 7, pp1394-1401.e4. "Consumption of fermented milk product with probiotic modulates brain activity."

257 Peter Andrey Smith for the *New York Times,* June 23, 2015. "Can the bacteria in your gut explain your mood?"

258 J Bravo, P Forsythe, et al. *PNAS.* 20 Sep 2011, vol. 108 no. 38, pp16050-5. "Ingestion of Lactobacillus strain regulates emotional behavior and central GABA receptor expression in a mouse via the vagus nerve."

259 J Alcock, C Maley, CA Aktipis. *Bioessays.* 2014 Oct; 36(10): 940-949. "Is eating behavior manipulated by the gastrointestinal microbiota? Evolutionary pressures and potential mechanisms."

260 Hawrelak JA, Myers SP. *Alternative Medicine Review.* 2004 Jun;9(2):180-97. "The causes of intestinal dysbiosis: a review."

261 Goehler LE, Gaykema RP, et al. *Brain, Behavior, and Immunology.* 2005 Jul;19(4):334-44. "Activation in vagal afferents and central autonomic pathways: early responses to intestinal infection with Campylobacter jejuni."

262 Baily MT, Coe CL. *Developmental Psychobiology.* 1999 Sep;35(2):146-55. "Maternal separation disrupts the integrity of the intestinal microflora in infant rhesus monkeys."

263 Liu S, Hagiwara SI, Bhargava A. *Neurogastroenterology and Motility.* 2017 Sep;29(9). "Early-life adversity, epigenetics, and visceral hypersensitivity."

264 Bercik P, Denou E, et al. *Gastroenterology.* 2011 Aug;141(2):599-609, 609.e1-3. "The intestinal microbiota affect central levels of brain-derived neurotropic factor and behavior in mice."

265 Amaral FA, Sachs D, et al. *PNAS.* 2008 Feb 12;105(6):2193-7. "Commensal microbiota is fundamental for the development of inflammatory pain."

266 J Alcock, C Maley, CA Aktipis. *Bioessays.* 2014 Oct; 36(10): 940-949. "Is eating behavior manipulated by the gastrointestinal microbiota? Evolutionary pressures and potential mechanisms."

267 David Kohn for *The Atlantic.* June 24, 2015. "When gut bacteria change brain function."

268 R Huang, K Wang, J Hu. *Nutrients.* 2016 Aug; 8(8): 483. "Effect of probiotics on depression: a systematic review and meta-analysis of randomized controlled trials."

269 Desbonnet L, Garrett L, et al. *Neuroscience.* 2010 Nov 10;170(4)1179-88. "Effects of the probiotic Bifidobacterium infantis in the maternal separation model of depression."

270 E Hsiao, S McBride, et al. *Cell.* 2013 Dec 19; 155(7): 1451-1463. "The microbiota modulates gut physiology and behavioral abnormalities associated with autism."

271 K Tillisch, J Labus, et al. *Gastroenterology.* 2013 Jun; 144(7): 10.1053/j. gastro.2013.02.043. "Consumption of fermented milk product with probiotic modulates brain activity."

272 J Bravo, P Forsythe, et al. *PNAS.* 20 Sep 2011, vol. 108 no. 38, pp16050-5. "Ingestion of Lactobacillus strain regulates emotional behavior and central GABA receptor expression in a mouse via the vagus nerve."

273 Benton D, Williams C, Brown A. *European Journal of Clinical Nutrition.* 2007 Mar;61(3):355-61. "Impact of consuming a milk drink containing a probiotic on mood and cognition."

274 Messaoudi M, Lalonde R, et al. *British Journal of Nutrition.* 2011 Mar;105(5):755-64. "Assessment of psychotropic-like properties of a probiotic formulation (L. helveticus R0052 and Bif longum R0175) in rats and human subjects."

275 Sawas T, Al Halabi S, et al. *Clinical Gastroenterology and Hepatology.* 2015 Sep;13(9):1567-74.e3. "Patients receiving prebiotics and probiotics before liver transplantation develop fewer infections than controls: A systematic review and mata-analysis."

276 Ritchie ML, Romanuk TN. *PLoS One.* 2012;7(4):e34938. "A meta-analysis of probiotic efficacy for gastrointestinal diseases."

277 Moayyedi P, Ford AC, et al. *Gut.* 2010 Mar;59(3):325-32. "The efficacy of probiotics in the treatment of irritable bowel syndrome: a systematic review."

278 Sinagra E, Morreale GC, et al. *World Journal of Gastroenterology.* 2017 Sep 28:23(36):6593-6627. "New therapeutic perspectives in IBS: targeting low-grade inflammation, immune-neuroendocrine axis, motility, secretion and beyond."

279 Didari T, Solki S, et al. *Expert Opinions on Drug Safety.* 2014 Feb;13(2):227-39. "A systematic review of the safety of probiotics."

280 Aaron E. Carroll for the *New York Times.* Oct 22, 2018. "The Problem with Probiotics."

281 J. Suez, N. Zmora, et al. *Cell.* 6 Sept 2018. 174(6): 1406-1423.e16. "Post-antibiotic gut mucosal microbiome reconstitution is impaired by probiotics and improved by autologous FMT."

282 David LA, Maurice CF, et al. *Nature.* 2014 Jan 23;505(7484):559-63. "Diet rapidly and reproducibly alters the human gut microbiome."

283 Wacklin P, Laurikka P, et al. *American Journal of Gastroenterology.* 2014 Dec;109(12):1933-41. "Altered duodenal microbiota composition in celiac disease patients suffering from persistent symptoms on a long-term gluten-free diet."

284 M Blaser. *Gastroenterology.* 2010 Dec; 139(6): 1819-1822. "Helicobacter pylori and esophageal disease: wake-up call?"

285 Wong RK, Yang C, et al. *Digestive Diseases and Sciences.* 2015 Jan;60(1):186-94. "Melatonin regulation as a possible mechanism for probiotic (VSL#3) in irritable bowel syndrome: a randomized double-blinded placebo study."

286 Ley RE, Turnbaugh PJ, et al. *Nature.* 2006 Dec 21;444(7122):1022-3. Microbial ecology: human gut microbes associated with obesity."

287 Turnbaugh PJ, Ley RE, et al. *Nature.* 2006 Dec 21;444(7122):1027-31. "An obesity-associated gut microbiome with increased capacity for energy harvest."

288 Summers RW, Elliott DE, et al. *Gut.* 2005 Jan;54(1):87-90. "Trichuris suis therapy in Crohn's disease."

289 Garg SK, Croft AM, Bager P. *Cochrane Database Systematic Review.* 2014 Jan 20;(1):CD009400. "Helminth therapy (worms) for induction of remission in inflammatory bowel disease."

290 T Kelesidis. *Therapeutic Advances in Gastroenterology.* 2012 Mar; 5(2): 111-125. "Efficacy and safety of the probiotic *Saccharomyces boulardii* for the prevention and therapy of gastrointestinal disorders."

291 Moré MI, Swidsinski A. *Clinical and Experimental Gastroenterology.* 2015 Aug 14;8:237-55. "Saccharomyces boulardii CNCM I-745 supports regeneration of the intestinal microbiota after diarrheic dysbiosis- a review.

292 Sonnenburg ED, Smits SA, et al. *Nature.* 2016 Jan 14;529(7585):212-5. "Diet-induced extinctions in the gut microbiota compound over generations."

293 S. El Aidy, T Dinan, J. Cryan. *Frontiers in Microbiology.* 2014; 5: 146. "Immune modulation of the brain-gut-microbe axis."

294 C de Lara, A Noble. *Biologics.* 2007 Jun; 1(2): 139-150. "Dishing the dirt on asthma: What we can learn from poor hygiene."

295 Olszak T, An D, et al. *Science.* 2012 Apr 27;336(6080):489-93. "Microbial exposure during early life has persistent effects on natural killer T cell function."

296 S Kinra, G Davey Smith, et al. *Thorax.* 2006 Jan; 61(1): 48-53. "Association between sibship size and allergic diseases in the Glasgow Alumni Study."

297 Adler A, Tager I, Quintero DR. *Journal of Allergy and Clinical Immunology.* 2005 Jan;115(1):67-73. "Decreased prevalence of asthma among farm-reared children compared with those who are rural but not farm-reared."

298 J Alcock, C Maley, CA Aktipis. *Bioessays.* 2014 Oct; 36(10): 940-949. "Is eating behavior manipulated by the gastrointestinal microbiota? Evolutionary pressures and potential mechanisms."

299 Zhang C, Yin A, et al. *EBioMedicine*. 2015 Jul 10;2(8):968-84. "Dietary modulation of gut microbiota contributes to alleviation of both genetic and simple obesity in children."

300 David Kohn for *The Atlantic*. June 24, 2015. "When gut bacteria change brain function."

301 Dr Robynne Chutkyne, *The Microbiome Solution: A Radical New Way to Heal Your Body from the Inside Out*. 1st edition August 2015, Avery.

302 T Kelesidis. *Therapeutic Advances in Gastroenterology*. 2012 Mar; 5(2): 111-125. "Efficacy and safety of the probiotic *Saccharomyces boulardii* for the prevention and therapy of gastrointestinal disorders."

303 Summers RW, Elliott DE, et al. *Gut*. 2005 Jan;54(1):87-90. "Trichuris suis therapy in Crohn's disease."

304 Julia Scott for the *New York Times Magazine*. May 22, 2014. "My No-Soap, No-Shampoo, Bacteria-Rich Hygeine Experiment."

305 Andrew Anthony for *The Guardian*. 11 February 2014. "I had the bacteria in my gut analyzed. And this may be the future of medicine."

306 Brian Handwerk for *National Geographic News*. March 26, 2013. "Once decimated U.S. fish stocks enjoy big bounce back."

307 Arthur Middleton in the *New York Times*. March 9, 2014. "Is the wolf a real American hero?"

308 Arthur Middleton in the NYT. March 9, 2014. "Is the wolf a real American hero?"

309 W Ripple, J Estes, et al. *Science*. 10 Jan 2014: Vol 343, Issue 6167, 1241484. "Status and ecological effects of the world's largest carnivores."

310 Heather Goldstone for WGBH News. Aug 6, 2014. "Could this be the end for Gulf of Maine cod?"

311 Teri Frady for National Oceanic and Atmospheric Association. Aug 1, 2014. "Statement Regarding New Information Showing Continued Decline of Gulf of Maine Cod Stock."

312 *The Economist*. May 27, 2017. "How to improve the health of the ocean."

313 *The Economist*. Feb 12, 2015. "Milking taxpayers. As crop prices fall, farmers grow subsidies instead."

314 Amelia Urry for *Grist*. April 20, 2015. "Our crazy farm subsidies, explained."

315 *The Wall Street Journal*. July 12, 2015. "Should Washington End Agriculture Subsidies?"

316 Marion Nestle for *Politico*. March 17, 2016. "The Farm Bill drove me insane."

317 Daniel Imhoff for *The Atlantic*. March 21, 2012. "Overhauling the Farm Bill: The real beneficiaries of subsidies."

318 James B Stewart for the *New York Times*. July 19, 2013. "Richer Farmers, Bigger Subsidies."

319 George Will in the *Washington Post*. June 7, 2013. "Sugar subsidies are immune to even modest reforms."

320 David Dayen in *The New Republic*. Feb 4, 2014. "The Farm Bill still gives wads of cash to agribusiness. It's just sneakier about it."

321 Jaclyn Moyer in *Salon*. Feb 9, 2015. "What nobody told me about small farming: I can't make a living."
Rebuttal:
The Ruminant, Feb 17, 2015. "'All Farmers Deserve to Make a Living!' Are we sure about that?"
Jaclyn Moyer (again) for *High Country News*. Dec 8, 2014. "When neighbors spray herbicides next to your organic crop."

322 G Feenstra, C Ingels, D Campbell, et al. UC Davis Sustainable Agriculture Institute, Research and Education Program. http://asi.ucdavis.edu/programs/sarep/about/what-is-sustainable-agriculture

323 D Pimentel, P Hepperly, et al. *BioScience*. Vol 55, Issue 7, 1 July 2005, pp 573-582. "Environmental, Energetic and Economic comparisons of organic and conventional farming systems." [Same title as a chapter by Pimentel D, Burges M. in 2014 book ed by Pimentel D and Peshin R "Integrated Pest Management. Springer, Dordrecht.]

324 Rodale Institute, Farming Systems Trial booklet/pdf: http://rodaleinstitute.org/assets/FSTbooklet.pdf

325 Chelsea Harvey for the *Washington Post*. Oct 17, 2016. "UN: Global agriculture needs a 'profound transformation' to fight climate change and protect food security."

326 Dan Charles for *NPR*'s *The Salt*. "Insects find a crack in biotech corn's armor."

327 Finamore A, Roselli M, et al. *Journal of Agriculture and Food Chemistry*. 2008 Dec 10;56(23):11533-9. "Intestinal and peripheral immune response to MON810 maize ingestion in weaning and old mice."

328 A Aris, S Leblanc. *Reproductive Toxicology*. 2011 May;31(4):528-33. "Maternal and fetal exposure to pesticides associated to genetically modified foods in eastern townships of Quebec, Canada."

329 R Raanan, K Harley, et al. *Environmental Health Perspectives.* 2015 Feb; 123(2): 179-185. "Early-life exposure to organophosphate pesticides and pediatric respiratory symptoms in the CHAMACOS cohort."

330 Raanan R, Balmes JR, et al. *Thorax.* 2016 Feb:71(2):148-53. "Decreased lung function in 7-year-old children with early-life organophosphate exposure"

331 P Grandjean, P Landrigan. *Lancet Neurology.* 2014 Mar; 13(3): 330-338. "Neurobehavioural effects of developmental toxicity."

332 Krüger M, Shehata AA, et al. *Anaerobe.* 2013 Apr;20:74-8. "Glyphosate suppresses the antagonistic effect of Enterococcus spp. on Clostridium botulinum."

333 Shehata AA, Schrödl W, et al. *Current Microbiology.* 2013 Apr;66(4):350-8. "The effect of glyphosate on potential pathogens and beneficial members of poultry microbiota in vitro."

334 Clair E, Linn L, et al. *Current Microbiology.* 2012 May;64(5):486-91. "Effects of Roundup and glyphosate on three food microorganisms: Geotrichum candidum, Lactococcus lactis subsp. cremoris and Lactobacillus delbrueckii subsp. bulgaricus."

335 Krüger M, Neuhaus J, et al. *Anaerobe.* 2014 Aug;28:220-5. "Chronic botulism in a Saxony dairy farm: sources, predisposing factors, development of the disease and treatment possibilities."

336 TERRIBLE study in 'Entropy' that needed an 'expression of concern' from the editors on glyphosate causing everything: A Samsel, S Seneff. Entropy. 2013, 15(4), 1416-1463. "Glyphosate's suppression of cytochrome P450 enzymes and amino acid biosynthesis by the gut microbiome: pathways to modern diseases."

337 Chiu YH, Williams PL, et al. *JAMA Internal Medicine.* 2018 Jan 1;178(1):17-26. "Association between pesticide residue intake from consumption of fruits and vegetables and pregnancy outcomes among women undergoing infertility treatment with assisted reproductive technology."

338 Kelsey Kopec and Lori Ann Burd for the Center for Biological Diversity. Feb 2017 Statement. "Pollinators in Peril: A systematic status review of North American and Hawaiian native bees."

339 AFP in *The Guardian.* 26 Feb 2016. "Decline of bees poses potential risks to major crops, says UN."

340 Union of Concerned Scientists GMO statement: http://www.ucsusa. org/our-work/food-agriculture/our-failing-food-system/genetic-engineering-agriculture#.VorrQs65fFI and American Academy of

Environmental Medicine GMO Statement: https://www.aaemonline. org/gmo.php

341 Jason Mark in *Scientific American*. Aug 14, 2011. "Myths: Busted— Clearing Up the Misunderstandings About Organic Farming."

342 Rodale Institute research page: http://rodaleinstitute.org/our-work/ research/

343 Mitchell AE, Hong YJ, et al. *Journal of Agriculture and Food Chemistry.* 2007 Jul 25;55(15):6154-9. "Ten-year comparison of the influence of organic and conventional crop management practices on the content of flavonoids in tomatoes."

344 G Butler, S Stergiadis, et el. *Journal of Dairy Science*. Jan 2011 vol 94 issue 1, pp 24-36. "Fat composition of organic and conventional retail milk in northeast England."

345 Reganold JP, Andrews PK, et al. *PLoS One.* 2010 Sep 1;5(9). pii: e12346. "Fruit and soil quality of organic and conventional strawberry agroecosystems."

346 NIH National Cancer Institute study on farm workers in Iowa ongoing since 1993: http://www.cancer.gov/about-cancer/causes-prevention/ risk/ahs-fact-sheet and website for updates: https://aghealth.nih.gov/

347 AR Bhat, MA Wani, et al. *Indian Journal of Medicine and Paediatric Oncology*. 2010 Oct-Dec; 31(4): 110-120. "Pesticides and brain cancer linked in orchard farmers of Kashmir."

348 Tom Philpott for *Mother Jones*. April 13, 2016. "Disturbing new evidence about what common pesticides can do to brains."

349 B Pearson, J Simin, et al. *Nature Communica*tions. 2016; 7: 11173. "Identification of chemicals that mimic transcriptional changes associated with autism, brain aging, and neurodegeneration."

350 Patrick Dolan from 1 Yard Revolution on their YouTube channel. "Why we don't use synthetic fertilizers." https://www.youtube.com/ watch?v=IxTHZ-hC9I0

351 AR Bhat, MA Wani, et al. *Indian Journal of Medicine and Paediatric Oncology*. 2010 Oct-Dec; 31(4): 110-120. "Pesticides and brain cancer linked in orchard farmers of Kashmir."

352 Jason Mark in *Scientific American*. Aug 14, 2011. "Myths: Busted— Clearing Up the Misunderstandings About Organic Farming."

353 Rodale Institute research page: http://rodaleinstitute.org/our-work/ research/

354 Antonio Roman-Alcalá for *Civil Eats*. April 19, 2016. "Can permaculture make a dent in America's farm landscape?"

355 *The Economist.* Feb 12, 2015. "Milking taxpayers. As crop prices fall, farmers grow subsidies instead." Amelia Urry for *Grist.* April 20, 2015. "Our crazy farm subsidies, explained." *The Wall Street Journal.* July 12, 2015. "Should Washington End Agriculture Subsidies?" Marion Nestle for *Politico.* March 17, 2016. "The Farm Bill drove me insane." Daniel Imhoff for *The Atlantic.* March 21, 2012. "Overhauling the Farm Bill: The real beneficiaries of subsidies." James B Stewart for the *New York Times.* July 19, 2013. "Richer Farmers, Bigger Subsidies." George Will in the *Washington Post.* June 7, 2013. "Sugar subsidies are immune to even modest reforms." David Dayen in the *New Republic.* Feb 4, 2014. "The Farm Bill still gives wads of cash to agribusiness. It's just sneakier about it."

356 Jaclyn Moyer in *Salon.* Feb 9, 2015. "What nobody told me about small farming: I can't make a living."
Rebuttal:
The Ruminant, Feb 17, 2015. "'All Farmers Deserve to Make a Living!' Are we sure about that?"
Jaclyn Moyer (again) for *High Country News.* Dec 8, 2014. "When neighbors spray herbicides next to your organic crop."

357 A Aris, S Leblanc. *Reproductive Toxicology.* 2011 May;31(4):528-33. "Maternal and fetal exposure to pesticides associated to genetically modified foods in eastern townships of Quebec, Canada."

358 Food and Agriculture Organization of the United Nations (FAO). "The State of Food and Agriculture 2014." http://www.fao.org/3/a-i4036e.pdf

359 D Pimentel, P Hepperly, et al. *BioScience.* Vol 55, Issue 7, 1 July 2005, pp 573-582. "Environmental, Energetic and Economic comparisons of organic and conventional farming systems." [Same title as a chapter by Pimentel D, Burges M. in 2014 book ed by Pimentel D and Peshin R "Integrated Pest Management. Springer, Dordrecht.]

360 Jason Mark in *Scientific American.* Aug 14, 2011. "Myths: Busted—Clearing Up the Misunderstandings About Organic Farming."

361 Tom Laskowy for *Grist.* July 22, 2011. "In defense of organic."

362 Tom Philpott for *Grist.* May 12, 2011. "Factory farms the only way to 'feed the world'? Not so, argues *Science* paper." Article cited: Reganold JP, Jackson-Smith D, et al. *Science.* 2011 May 6;332(6030):670-1. "Agriculture. Transforming U.S. agriculture." and newer article: Crowder DW, Reganold JP. *PNAS.* 2015 Jun 16;112(24):7611-6. "Financial competitiveness of organic agriculture on a global scale."

363 D Pimentel, P Hepperly, et al. *BioScience.* Vol 55, Issue 7, 1 July 2005, pp 573-582. "Environmental, Energetic and Economic comparisons of organic and conventional farming systems." [Same title as a chapter by Pimentel D, Burges M. in 2014 book ed by Pimentel D and Peshin R "Integrated Pest Management. Springer, Dordrecht.]

364 Union of Concerned Scientists GMO statement: http://www.ucsusa. org/our-work/food-agriculture/our-failing-food-system/genetic-engineering-agriculture#.VorrQs65fFI and American Academy of Environmental Medicine GMO Statement: https://www.aaemonline. org/gmo.php

365 L Hunter Lovins in *The Guardian Sustainable Business.* 19 August 2014. "Why George Monbiot is wrong: grazing livestock can save the world."

366 Gregory Barber for *Mother Jones.* Feb 10, 2016. "Are cage-free eggs all they're cracked up to be?"

367 *Perennial Plate* series: http://www.theperennialplate.com/.

368 National Research Council, Board on Agriculture and Natural Resources, Institute of Medicine, Food and Nutrition Board. "Planning Committee on Exploring the True Costs of Food: A Workshop. Chapter 2: Exploring Health and Environmental Costs of Food: Workshop Summary." National Academies Press (US); 2012 Dec 28. http://www.ncbi.nlm.nih.gov/books/NBK236855/.

369 G Keoleian, D Przybylo. University of Michigan Center for Sustainable Systems. 2010. "Full Life Cycle Costs of Organic vs Conventional Food." (updated fact sheet: http://css.umich.edu/ factsheets/us-food-system-factsheet)

370 Hannah Wallace for *Modern Farmer.* Jan 6, 2016. "Uncle Sam makes it easier for your SNAP benefits to go toward a CSA share."

371 Jo Robinson, *Eating on the Wild Side.* Little, Brown and Company; 1 edition June 4, 2013.

372 Daphne Miller, M.D. *The Jungle Effect.* Published by William Morrow 4/08.

373 Dan Buettner. The Blue Zones Solution: Eating and Living Like the World's Healthiest People. *National Geographic*, April 2015.

374 Planting Justice: San Francisco Bay area since 2009. http://www. plantingjustice.org

375 St Louis MetroMarket: St. Louis mobile farmers market serving food deserts since 2015. https://www.stlmetromarket.com/

376 Kim Willsher for *The Guardian*. 10 December 2015. "French MPs vote to force supermarkets to give away unsold food"

377 Growing Power: Milwaukee organization to teach urban farming, 1995-2017.

378 Green Veterans (via the US Green Building Council): Helping vets make the military to civilian transition with green entrepreneurship, sustainable building and green living.

379 Victory Garden Initiative: Milwaukee organization dedicated to improving food security through teaching gardening since 2013. http://victorygardeninitiative.org

380 The Grange School of Adaptive Agriculture, Mendocino County: 14-week vocational residential agriculture training program teaching the science, art, and business of food. http://www.school-of-adaptive-agriculture.org/

381 Victory Greens at Lennox Hill Hospital and Harlem Grown in NYC: improving food access with microfarms and education for youth. http://jobs.northwell.edu/blog/2017/06/26/victory-greens-lenox-hill/

382 A Zumkehr, JE Campbell. *Frontiers in Ecology and the Environment*. 1 June 2015, 13:244-248. "The potential for local croplands to meet US food demand."

383 Mark Bittman, Michael Pollan, Ricardo Salvador, and Olivier De Schutter in the *Washington Post*. Nov 7, 2014. "How a national food policy could save millions of American lives."

384 Steve Holt for *Civil Eats*. Nov 10, 2015. "Does U.S. Farm Policy Have a Race Problem?"

385 Cliff Weathers in *Salon*. March 14, 2015. "Bottled water is a scam: PepsiCo, Coca-Cola and the beverage industry's greatest con."

386 Alexandra Sifferlin for *Time*. April 18, 2017. "Do soda taxes really work?"

387 Allison Aubrey for *NPR*'s *The Salt*. Oct 11, 2016. "Tax soda to fight obesity, WHO urges nations around the globe."

388 Allison Aubrey for *NPR*'s *The Salt*. Oct 20, 2016. "Trick or treat? Critics blast big soda's efforts to fend off taxes."

389 Pearson-Stuttard J, Bandosz P, et al. *PLoS Medicine*. 2017 Jun 6;14(6):e1002311. "Reducing US cardiovascular disease burden and disparities through national and targeted dietary policies: A modeling study."

390 Brigid Schulte for the *Washington Post*. June 2, 2015. "Health experts have figured out how much time you should sit each day."

391 Thompson Coon J, Boddy K, et al. *Environment, Science, and Technology.* 2011 Mar 1;45(5):1761-72. "Does participating in physical activity in outdoor natural environments have a greater effect on physical and mental wellbeing than physical activity indoors? A systematic review."

392 R. Mitchell. *Social Science and Medicine.* 2013 Aug;91:130-4. "Is physical activity in natural environments better for mental health than physical activity in other environments?"

393 J Barton, J Pretty. *Environmental Science and Technology.* 2010, 44(10), pp3947-3955. "What is the best dose of nature and green exercise for improving mental health? A multi-study analysis."

394 Pfotenhauer KM, Shubrook JH. *Journal of the American Osteopathic Association.* 2017 May 1;117(5):301-305. "Vitamin D deficiency, its role in health and disease, and current supplementation recommendations."

395 Mortimer JA, Ding D, et al. *Journal of Alzheimers Disease.* 2012;30(4):757-66. "Changes in brain volume and cognition in a randomized trial of exercise and social interaction in a community-based sample of non-demented Chinese elders."

396 Colombe SJ, Erickson KI, et al. *Journal of Geronology, Biological Sciences and Medical Sciences Series A.* 2006 Nov;61(11):1166-70. "Aerobic exercise training increases brain volume in aging humans."

397 Uusi-Rasi K, Patil R. et al. *JAMA Internal Medicine.* 2015 May;175(5):703-11. "Exercise and vitamin D in fall prevention among older women: a randomized clinical trial."

398 F. Li, P Harmer, et al. *JAMA Internal Medicine.* 2018 Oct;178(10):1301-1310. "Effectiveness of a Therapeutic Tai Ji Quan Intervention vs a Multimodal Exercise Intervention to Prevent Falls Among Older Adults at High Risk of Falling"

399 C. Lunghi, Sale A. *Current Biology.* Volume 25, Issue 23, pR1122-3, 7 Dec 2015. "A cycling lane for brain rewiring."

400 *Epigenetics* 2014 Dec;9(12):1557-69. "An integrative analysis reveals coordinated reprogramming of the epigenome and the transcriptome in human skeletal muscle after training."

401 Olga Khazan for *The Atlantic.* March 24, 2014. "For Depression, Prescribing Exercise Before Medication."

402 D Bavelier, CS Green, et al. *Nature Reviews Neuroscience.* 2011 Dec; 12(12): 763-768. "Brains on video games."

403 Grover K, Pecor K, et al. *Journal of Child Neurology.* 2016 Jun;31(7):850-7. "Effects of instant messaging on school performance in adolescents."

404 "#Being Thirteen: Social Media and the Hidden World of Young Adolescents' Peer Culture." M Underwood, R Faris. Collaboration with CNN, and Anderson Cooper 360. https://www.documentcloud. org/documents/2448422-being-13-report.html and related Oct 13, 2015 CNN article by Chuck Hadad: "Why some 13-year-olds check social media 100 times a day."

405 Pew Research Center study by Amanda Lenhart. April 9, 2015. "Teens, Social Media & Technology Overview 2015."

406 Biswas A, Oh PI, et al. *Annals of Internal Medicine.* 2015 Jan 20;162(2):123-32. "Sedentary time and its association with risk for disease incidence, mortality, and hospitalization in adults: a systematic review and meta-analysis."

407 Shen D, Mao W, et al. *PLoS One.* 2014; 9(8): e105709. "Sedentary behavior and incident cancer: A meta-analysis of prospective studies."

408 Wilmot EG, Edwardson CL, et al. *Diabetologia.* 2012 Nov;55(11);2895-905. "Sedentary time in adults and the association with diabetes, cardiovascular disease and death: systematic review and meta-analysis."

409 Patel AV, Bernstein L, et al. *American Journal of Epidemiology.* 2010 Aug 15;172(4):419-29. "Leisure time spending sitting in relation to total mortality in a prospective cohort of US adults."

410 Henson J, Davies MJ, et al. *Diabetes Care.* 2016 Jan;39(1):130-8. "Breaking up prolonged sitting with standing or walking attenuates the postprandial metabolic response in postmenopausal women: A randomized acute study."

411 Diana Swift for *Medscape.* June 2, 2015. "Desk workers should stand, walk 2 hours during workday." *British Journal of Sports Medicine* Consensus Statement. June 17, 2015. "The sedentary office: a growing case for change towards better health and productivity. Expert statement commissioned by Public Health England and the Active Working Community Interest Company." http://bjsm.bmj.com/content/early/2015/04/23/bjsports-2015-094618.full

412 S Colberg, R Sigal, et al. *Diabetes Care Journal.* 2016 Nov;29(11): 2065-2079. "Physical Activity/Exercise and Diabetes: A position statement of the American Diabetes Association."

413 Lauby-Secretan B, Scoccianti C, et al. *New England Journal of Medicine.* 2016 Aug 25;375(8):794-8. "Body Fatness and Cancer—Viewpoint of the IARC Working Group."

414 Högström G, Nordström A, Nordström P. *International Journal of Epidemiology.* 2016 Aug;45(4):1159-1168. "Aerobic fitness in late

adolescence and the risk of early death: a prospective cohort study of 1.3 million Swedish men."

415 Caleyachetty R, Thomas GN, et al. *Journal of American College of Cardiology.* 2017 Sep 19;70(12):1429-1437. "Metabolically healthy obese and incident cardiovascular disease events among 3.5 million men and women."

416 Nicola Twilley and Cynthia Graber from *Gastropod*, for digg.com, Jan 26, 2016. "The calorie is broken. It's time to burn it."

417 Scott Cuyjet for *Journal Watch*: In Practice. March 2, 2016. "Think Outside the Scale."

418 T Wang, Y Heianza, et al. *British Medical Journal.* 2018; 360: j5644. "Improving adherence to healthy dietary patterns, genetic risk, and long term weight gain: gene-diet interaction analysis in two prospective cohort studies."

419 D Lee, R Pate, et al. *Journal of the American College of Cardiology.* 2014 Aug 5; 64(5): 472-481. "Leisure-time running reduces all-cause and cardiovascular mortality risk."

420 A Wong, A Figueroa, et al. *Menopause.* 2018 Feb 12 doi: 10.1097/GME.0000000000001072. "The effects of stair climbing on arterial stiffness, blood pressure, and leg strength in postmenopausal women with stage 2 hypertension."

421 Ross R, Hudson R, et al. *Annals of Internal Medicine.* 2015 Mar 3;162(5):325-34. "Effects of exercise amount and intensity on abdominal obesity and glucose tolerance in obese adults: a randomized trial."

422 Centers for Disease Control and Prevention (CDC) exercise guidelines: http://www.cdc.gov/physicalactivity/basics/adults/index.htm

423 Arem H, Moore SC, et al. *JAMA Internal Medicine.* 2015 Jun;175(6):959-67. "Leisure time physical activity and mortality: a detailed pooled analysis of the dose-response relationship."

424 Arem H, Moore SC, et al. *JAMA Internal Medicine.* 2015 Jun;175(6):959-67. "Leisure time physical activity and mortality: a detailed pooled analysis of the dose-response relationship."

425 Hupin D, Roche F, et al. *British Journal of Sports Medicine.* 2015 Oct;49(19):1262-7. "Even a low-dose of moderate-to-vigorous physical activity reduces mortality by 22 percent in adults aged > 60 years: a systematic review and meta-analysis."

426 Gillen JB, Percival ME, et al. *PLoS One.* 2014 Nov 3;9(11):e111489. "Three minutes of all-out intermittent exercise per week increases

skeletal muscle oxidative capacity and improves cardiometabolic health."

427 Gretchen Reynolds for the *New York Times*. Dec 10, 2014. "Got a minute? Let's work out." http://well.blogs.nytimes.com/2014/12/10/one-minute-workout/

428 Gliemann L, Gunnarsson TP, et al. *Scandinavian Journal of Medicine Science and Sports*. 2015 Oct;25(5):e479-89. "10-20-30 training increases performance and lowers blood pressure and VEGF in runners."

429 *Epigenetics* 2014 Dec;9(12):1557-69. "An integrative analysis reveals coordinated reprogramming of the epigenome and the transcriptome in human skeletal muscle after training."

430 Diana Swift for *Medscape*. June 2, 2015. "Desk workers should stand, walk 2 hours during workday."

431 *British Journal of Sports Medicine* Consensus Statement. June 17, 2015. "The sedentary office: a growing case for change towards better health and productivity. Expert statement commissioned by Public Health England and the Active Working Community Interest Company." http://bjsm.bmj.com/content/early/2015/04/23/bjsports-2015-094618.full

432 Gillespie LD, Robertson MC, et al. *Cochrane Database Systemic Review*. 2009 Apr 15;(2): CD007146. "Interventions for preventing falls in older people living in the community."

433 Sharon Begley for *Time*. Jan 19, 2007. "The brain: How the brain rewires itself. Not only can the brain learn new tricks, but it can also change its structure and function—even in old age."

434 Tooley GA, Armstrong SM, et al. *Biological Psychology*. 2000 May;53(1):69-78. "Acute increases in night-time plasma melatonin levels following a period of meditation."

435 R. Nagendra, N. Maruthai, B. Kutty. *Frontiers in Neurology*. 2012; 3: 54. "Meditation and its regulatory role on sleep."

436 Black DS, O'Reilly GA, et al. *JAMA Internal Medicine*. 2015 Apr;175(4):494-501. "Mindfulness meditation and improvement in sleep quality and daytime impairment among older adults with sleep disturbances: a randomized clinical trial."

437 Davidson RJ, Kabat-Zinn J, et al. *Psychosomatic Medicine*. 2003 Jul-Aug;65(4):564-70. "Alterations in brain and immune function produced by mindfulness meditation."

438 J. Dusek, H. Otu, et al. *PLOS One.* July 2, 2008. "Genomic Counter-Stress Changes Induced by the Relaxation Response."

439 Barrett B, Hayney MS, et al. *Annals of Family Medicine.* 2012 Jul-Aug;10(4):337-46. "Meditation or exercise for preventing acute respiratory infection: a randomized controlled trial"

440 Ornish D, Magbanua MJ, et al. *PNAS.* 2008 Un 17;105(24):8369-74. "Changes in prostate gene expression in men undergoing an intensive nutrition and lifestyle intervention."

441 Carlson LE, Beattie TL, et al. *Cancer.* 2015 Feb 1;121(3):476-84. "Mindfullness-based cancer recovery and supportive-expressive therapy maintain telomere length relative to controls in distressed breast cancer survivors."

442 Carlson LE, Tamagawa R, et al. *Psychooncology.* 2016 Jul:25(7):750-9. "Raondomized-controlled trial of mindfulness-based cancer recovery versus supportive expressive group therapy among distressed breast cancer survivors (MINDSET): long-term follow-up results."

443 Bhasin MK, Dusek JA, et al. *PLoS One.* 2013 May 1;8(5):e62817. "Relaxation response induces temporal transcriptome changes in energy metabolism, insulin secretion and inflammatory pathways."

444 Florence Williams for *National Geographic.* Jan 2016. "This is your brain on nature."

445 UMASS Medical School Center for Mindfulness in Medicine, Health Care, and Society. Research on MBSR: http://umassmed.edu/cfm/research/publications/

446 NIH research search page with keyword "mindfulness" http://search.nih.gov/search?utf8=√&affiliate=nih&query=mindfulness&commit.x=0&commit.y=0&commit=Search

447 B Hölzel, J Carmody, et al. *Psychiatry Research.* 2011 Jan 30; 191(1): 36-43. "Mindfulness practice leads to increases in regional brain grey matter density."

448 Kaliman P, Alvarez-López JM, et al. *Psychoneuroendocrinology.* 2014 Feb;40:96-107. "Rapid changes in histone deacetylases and inflammatory gene expression in expert meditators."

449 Mata D, Ramos M, et al. *JAMA.* 2015;314(22):2373-2383. "Prevalence of depression and depressive symptoms among resident physicians."

450 Natalie Goldberg *The great spring: writing, zen, and this zigzag life.* Shambala, February 2016.

451 Logan AC, Selhub EM. *Biophychosocial Medicine.* 2012 Apr 3;6(1):11. "Vis medicatrix naturae: does nature 'minister to the mind'?"

452 Raymond De Young "Environmental Psychology Overview" Ch 2, pp 17-33 in *Green Organizations: Driving change with I-O psychology*. Ann Hergatt Huffman, Stephanie R Klein eds. 2013 Taylor & Francis.

453 James Hamblin for *The Atlantic*. Oct 2015. "The Nature Cure. Why some doctors are writing prescriptions for time outdoors." (ecotherapy with references)

454 R Berto. *Behavioral Science*. 2014 Dec; 4(4):394-409. "The role of nature in coping with psycho-physiological stress: literature review on restorativeness."

455 Amoly E, Dadvand P, et al. *Environmental Health Perspectives*. 2014 Dec;122(12):1351-8. "Green and blue spaces and behavioral development in Barcelona schoolchildren: the BREATHE project."

456 J Craig, A Logan, S Prescott. *Journal of Physiological Anthropology*. 2016; 35: 1. "Natural environments, nature relatedness and the ecological theater: connecting satellites and sequencing to shinrin-yoku."

457 Kronholm E, Puusniekka R, et al. *Journal of Sleep Research*. 2015 Feb;24(1):3-10. "Trends in self-reported sleep problems, tiredness and related school performance among Finnish adolescents from 1984-2011." (particularly interesting since Finns have the best school performance of all countries)

458 D Bavelier, CS Green, et al. *Nature Reviews Neuroscience*. 2011 Dec; 12(12): 763-768. "Brains on video games."

459 Grover K, Pecor K, et al. *Journal of Child Neurology*. 2016 Jun;31(7):850-7. "Effects of instant messaging on school performance in adolescents."

460 (same study). Pecor K, Kang L, et al. *Brain Development*. 2016 Jun;38(6):548-53. "Sleep health, messaging, headaches, and academic performance in high school students."

461 "#Being Thirteen: Social Media and the Hidden World of Young Adolescents' Peer Culture." M Underwood, R Faris. Collaboration with CNN, and Anderson Cooper 360. https://www.documentcloud. org/documents/2448422-being-13-report.html and related Oct 13, 2015 CNN article by Chuck Hadad: "Why some 13-year-olds check social media 100 times a day."

462 Pew Research Center study by Amanda Lenhart. April 9, 2015. "Teens, Social Media & Technology Overview 2015."

463 Clark L, Rhea D. *International Journal of Child Health and Nutrition*. May 2017, vol 6, pp 54-61. "The LiiNK Project: Comparisons of recess, physical activity, and positive emotional states in grade K-2 children."

464 N Seltenrich. *Environmental Health Perspectives*. 2015 Oct; 123(10): A254-259. "Just what the doctor ordered: using parks to improve children's health."

465 Maas J, Verheij RA, et al. *Journal of Epidemiology and Community Health*. 2009 Dec;63(12):967-73. "Morbidity is related to a green living environment."

466 Kabisch N, van den Bosch M, Lafortezza R. *Environmental Research*. 2017 Nov;159:362-373. "The health benefits of nature-based solutions to urbanization challenges for children and the elderly- A systematic review."

467 F Kuo, A Faber Taylor. *American Journal of Public Health*. 2004 September; 94(9): 1580-1586. "A potential natural treatment for attention-deficit disorder: evidence from a national study."

468 Largo-Wight E. *International Journal of Environmental Health Research*. "cultivating healthy places and communities: evidence-based nature contact recommendations."

469 S Warber, A DeHudy, et al. *Evidence Based Complementary and Alternative Medicine*. 2015; 2015: 651827. "Addressing 'Nature-Deficit disorder': a mixed methods pilot study of young adults attending a wilderness camp."

470 Park BJ, Tsunetsugu Y, et al. *Environmental Health and Preventative Medicine*. 2010 Jan;15(1):18-26. "The physiological effects of Shinrin-yoku (taking in the forest atmosphere or forest bathing) evidence from field experiments in 24 forests across Japan."

471 Song C, Ikei H, Miyazaki Y. *International Journal of Environmental Research and Public Health*. 2016 Aug 3;13(8). "Physiological effects of nature therapy: a review of the research in Japan."

472 Cho KS, Lim YR, et al. *Toxicology Research*. 2017 Apr;33(2):97-106. "Terpenes from forests and human health."

473 Reid KJ, Santostasi G, et al. *PLoS One*. 2014 Apr 2;9(4):e92251. "Timing and Intensity of Light Correlate with Body Weight in Adults."

474 Roenneberg T, Allegrandt KV, et al. *Current Biology*. 2012 May 22;22(10):939-43. "Social jetlag and obesity."

475 H Christensen, P Batterham, et al. *The Lancet Psychiatry*. 2016 Apr;3(4):333-41. "Effectiveness of an online insomnia program (SHUTi) for prevention of depressive episodes (the GoodNight study): a randomized controlled trial."

476 C Coutts, M Hahn. *International Journal of Environmental Research and Public Health*. 2015 Aug; 12(8): 9768-9798. "Green infrastructure, ecosystem services, and Human Health."

477 David Crouch for *The Guardian*. 17 September 2015. "Efficiency up, turnover down: Sweden experiments with six-hour working day."

478 John Pencavel, 9 Oct 2014, *The Economic Journal*, vol 125, issue 589, pp2052-2076. "The productivity of working hours."

479 C.W. in *The Economist*. Dec 9, 2014. "Proof that you should get a life."

480 Atul Gawande, *Being Mortal: Medicine and what matters in the end*. 2014 Picador.

481 Pagidipati NJ, Navar AM, et al. *JAMA*. 2017 Apr 18;317(15):1563-1567. "Comparison of recommended eligibility for primary prevention statin therapy based on the US preventive services task force recommendations vs the ACC/AHA guidelines."

482 David Epstein and ProPublica in *The Atlantic*. Feb 22, 2017. "When evidence says no, but doctors say yes."

483 Vinayak Prasad, Adam Cifu, *Ending Medical Reversal: Improving outcomes, saving lives*. 2015 Johns Hopkins University Press.

484 Victoria Sweet, *God's Hotel: a doctor, a hospital, and a pilgrimage to the heart of medicine*. 2012 Riverhead.

485 Sonnenburg ED, Smits SA, et al. *Nature*. 2016 Jan 14;529(7585):212-5. "Diet-induced extinctions in the gut microbiota compound over generations."

486 N Wilck, MG Matus, et al. *Nature*. 2017 Nov 30;551(7682):585-589. "Salt-responsive gut commensal modulates TH17 axis and disease."

487 Boyer J, Liu RH. *Nutrition*. 2004; 3:5. "Apple phytochemicals and their health benefits."

488 Hill CL, March LM, et al. *Annals of Rheumatological Diseases*. 2016 Jan;75(1):23-9. "Fish oil in knee osteoarthritis: a randomized clinical trial of low dose versus high dose."

489 Tom Phillpott for *Mother Jones*, Feb 3, 2016. "WTF happened to golden rice?"

490 Stevens G, Bennett J, et al. *The Lancet*. 2015 Sep;3(9):e528-36. "Trends and mortality effects of vitamin A deficiency in children in 138 low-income and middle-income countries between 1991 and 2013: a pooled analysis of population-based surveys."

491 Qato DM, Wilder J, et al. *JAMA Internal Medicine*. 2016 Apr;176(4):473-82. "Changes in prescription and over-the-counter

medication and dietary supplement use among older adults in the United States, 2005-2011.

492 S Cummings, D Kiel, D Black. *JAMA Internal Medicine*, Editorial. 2016 Feb;176(2):171-172. "Vitamin D supplementation and increased risk of falling: A cautionary tale of vitamin supplements retold."

493 Bischoff-Ferrari HA, Dawson-Hughes B, et al. *JAMA Internal Medicine*. 2016 Feb;176(2):175-83. "Monthly high-dose vitamin D treatment for the prevention of functional decline: a randomized clinical trial."

494 Nathaniel Rich in *New York Times Magazine*. Jan 6, 2016. "The lawyer who became DuPont's worst nightmare."

495 K Maresz. *Integrative Medicine*. 2015 Feb; 14(1): 34-39. Proper Calcium Use: Vitamin K2 as a promoter of bone and cardiovascular health."

496 Zheng H, Yde CC, et al. *Journal of Agriculture and Food Chemistry*. 2015 Mar 18;63(10):2830-9. "Metabolomics investigation to shed light on cheese as a possible piece in the French paradox puzzle."

497 Bischoff-Ferrari HA, Dawson-Hughes B, et al. *JAMA Internal Medicine*. 2016 Feb;176(2):175-83. "Monthly high-dose vitamin D treatment for the prevention of functional decline: a randomized clinical trial."

498 Gonçalves R, Lourenço A, Silva SN. *International Journal of Drug Policy*. 2015 Feb;26(2):199-209. "A social cost perspective in the wake of the Portuguese strategy for the fight against drugs."

499 Rog DJ, Marshall T, et al. *Psychiatric Services*. 2014 Mar 1;65(3):287-94. "Permanent supportive housing: assessing the evidence."

500 Aubry T, Nelson G, Tsemberis S. *Canadian Journal of Psychiatry*. 2015 Nov;60(11):467-74. "Housing first for people with severe mental illness who are homeless: a review of the research and findings from the At Home-Chez soi demonstration project."

501 Mackelprang JL, Collins SE, Clifasefi SL. *Prehospital Emergency Care*. 2014 Oct-Dec;18(4):476-82. "Housing first is associated with reduced use of emergency medical services."

502 Jo Marchant, *CURE*. 2016, Crown.

503 A Sekar, A Bialas, et al. *Nature*. 2016 Feb 11;530(7589): 177-183. "Schizophrenia risk from complex variation of complement component 4."

504 C Kinch, K Ibhazehiebo, et al. *PNAS*. 2015 Feb 3; 112(5): 1475-1480. "Low-dose exposure to bisphenol A and replacement bisphenol

S induces precocious hypothalamic neurogenesis in embryonic zebrafish."

505 D Mata, M Ramos, et al. *JAMA*. 2015 Dec 8; 314(22): 2373-2383. "Prevalence of depression and depressive symptoms among resident physicians a systemic review and meta-analysis."

506 *MedPage Today* (Staff Writer), Sept 25, 2016. "Half of physicians demoralized dissatisfied- Survey: job dissatisfaction rampant in medicine."

507 Atul Gawande, *Being Mortal: Medicine and what matters in the end*. 2014 Picador.

508 Lisa Krieger in *The Mercury News*. Feb 5, 2012. "The cost of dying: It's hard to reject care even as costs soar."

509 Ken Murray in *Zócalo*. "How Doctors Die: It's not like the rest of us, but it should be."

510 Laura Selby in *The DO*. Sept 11, 2015. "OMT, pureed carrots and immersion: Teaching students end-of life care."

511 *NPR Morning Edition* interview: Dr Lucy Kalanithi about her late husband Dr Paul Kalanithi's book "Inside a doctor's mind at the end of his life. Feb 12, 2016. [*When Breath Becomes Air*. Random House 2016.]

512 *The Economist*, Apr 29, 2017 "How to have a better death: Death is inevitable. A bad death is not."

513 Atul Gawande, *Being Mortal: Medicine and what matters in the end*. 2014 Picador. 4 questions from Epilogue p 259.

514 David Cumes, *The Source: The story of an indigenous healing center in remote South Africa*. Aug 2017.

515 Zen Hospice Project website: http://www.zenhospice.org

516 Dhruv Khullar, the *New York Times*, "How Behavioral Economics Can Produce Better Health Care." April 13, 2017.

517 E. Brandt, R. Myerson, M Coca Perraillon, "Hospital Admissions for MI and CVA Before and After the Trans-Fatty Acid Restrictions in New York." *JAMA Cardiology* 2017;2(6):627-634.

518 Dan Buettner. The Blue Zones Solution: Eating and Living Like the World's Healthiest People. *National Geographic*, April 2015.

519 M Springman, HC Godfray, et al. *Proceedings of the National Academy of Sciences*. April 12, 2016, vol 113 no 15 p 4146-4151. "Analysis and valuation of the health and climate change cobenefits of dietary change."

520 DL Katz, S Meller. *Annual Review of Public Health.* Vol. 35:83-103. March 2014. "Can we say what diet is best for health?"

521 Valls-Pedret C, Sala-Vila A, et al. *JAMA Internal Medicine.* 2015 Jul;175(7):1094-103. "Mediterranean diet and age-related cognitive decline: a randomized clinical trial."

522 Dan Buettner. The Blue Zones Solution: Eating and Living Like the World's Healthiest People. *National Geographic,* April 2015.

523 M.S.L.J. for *The Economist.* April 19, 2016. "Why eating more vegetables is good for the environment."

524 Staudacher HM. *Journal of Gastroenterology and Hepatology.* 2017 Mar;32 Suppl 1:16-19. "Nutritional, microbiological and psychosocial implications of the low FODMAP diet.

525 Jerry Adler for *The Smithsonian.* June 2013. "Why Fire Makes Us Human."

526 D Ornish, SE Brown, et al. *The Lancet.* 21 July 1990. Vol 336, No. 8708, p129-133. "Can lifestyle changes reverse coronary heart disease? The Lifestyle Heart Trial."

527 Shai I, Spense JD, et al. *Circulation.* 2010 Mar 16;121(10):1200-8. "Dietary intervention to reverse carotid atherosclerosis."

528 Peter Whoriskey for the *Washington Post.* May 1, 2017. "Why your 'organic' milk may not be organic."

529 RM Anson, Z Guo, et al. *PNAS.* 13 May 2003, vol 100 no. 10, p6216-6220. "Intermittent fasting dissociates beneficial effects of dietary restriction on glucose metabolism and neuronal resistance to injury from calorie intake." (M. Mattson)

530 B Martin, M Mattson, S Maudsley. *Ageing Research Review.* 2006 Aug; 5(3): 332-353. "Caloric restriction and intermittent fasting: Two potential diets for successful brain aging."

531 M Maalouf, J Rho, M Mattson. *Brain Research Review.* 2009 Mar; 59(2): 293-315. "The neuroprotective properties of calorie restriction, the ketogenic diet, and ketone bodies."

532 Zarrinpar A, Chaix A, et al. *Cell Metabolism.* 2014 Dec 2;20(6):1006-17. "Diet and feeding pattern affect the diurnal dynamics of the gut microbiome."

533 S Brandhorst, IY Choi, et al. *Cell Metabolism.* 2015 Jul 7;22(1):86-99. "A periodic diet that mimics fasting promotes multi-system regeneration, enhanced cognitive performance, and healthspan." (V. Longo) (1090 cal day 1 then 2-5 725) http://www.cell.com/cell-metabolism/fulltext/S1550-4131(15)00224-7

534 J Trepanowski, C Kroeger, et al. *JAMA Internal Medicine.* 2017;177(7):930-938. "Effect of alternate-day fasting on weight loss, weight maintenance, and cardioprotection among metabolically healthy obese adults. A randomized clinical trial."

535 S. Furmli, R. Elmasry, et al. *BMJ Case Reports* 2018; doi: 10.1136/bcr-2017-221854 "Therapeutic use of intermittent fasting for people with type 2 diabetes as an alternative to insulin."

536 DL Katz, S Meller. *Annual Review of Public Health.* March 2014 Vol 35:83-103. "Can we say what diet is best for health?"

CPSIA information can be obtained
at www.ICGtesting.com
Printed in the USA
BVHW031057100519
547846BV00022B/87/P